SERVICE YOUR
SMILE

SERVICE YOUR SMILE

How Orthodontic Treatment Can **Change Your Life**

Ara Agopian DDS, MS

Published by Advantage, Charleston, South Carolina.
Member of Advantage Media Group.

ADVANTAGE is a registered trademark, and the Advantage colophon is a trademark of Advantage Media Group, Inc.

Printed in the United States of America.

10 9 8 7 6 5 4 3 2 1

ISBN: 978-1-59932-991-8
LCCN: 2018953932

Cover design by Mary Hamilton.
Layout design by Wesley Strickland.

This publication is designed to provide accurate and authoritative information in regard to the subject matter covered. It is sold with the understanding that the publisher is not engaged in rendering legal, accounting, or other professional services. If legal advice or other expert assistance is required, the services of a competent professional person should be sought.

 Advantage Media Group is proud to be a part of the Tree Neutral® program. Tree Neutral offsets the number of trees consumed in the production and printing of this book by taking proactive steps such as planting trees in direct proportion to the number of trees used to print books. To learn more about Tree Neutral, please visit **www.treeneutral.com**.

Advantage Media Group is a publisher of business, self-improvement, and professional development books and online learning. We help entrepreneurs, business leaders, and professionals share their Stories, Passion, and Knowledge to help others Learn & Grow. Do you have a manuscript or book idea that you would like us to consider for publishing? Please visit **advantagefamily.com** or call **1.866.775.1696**.

Table of Contents

Part One: A Category of One

Part Two: Your Mouth at Every Age

Part One

A Category of One

Introduction

I spent the first years of my life in Beirut, Lebanon, a war-torn country that has been in turmoil for decades. I completed high school amidst the country's conflicts and civil wars.

Growing up, I only went to the dentist when something hurt—when a new cavity had appeared or a tooth ached. Most dentists everywhere know that when something hurts, it's already too late. Unfortunately, dental care and hygiene were not important in Lebanon. My family dentist never once gave me any type of preventive instructions to avoid cavities or decay. We were not taught the importance of daily flossing and brushing; it was all drill and fill.

By the time I was nineteen, I had experienced a few root canals and donned a few crowns. I didn't realize how poor the dental care really was until I immigrated to the United States.

I came to the United States as a student and initially settled in Los Angeles. Only two months into my first semester in college, I knew finances would be an issue. My family did not have the financial means to support a student abroad. Unfortunately, the scholarship and financial assistance I was counting on did not come through and I could not afford it all. I received tuition notices in my mailbox, stating to pay or be kicked out, so I chose the latter and dropped out of school.

In order to avoid becoming an undocumented immigrant, I left the United States. At the time, Canada was accepting refugees from war-torn countries, including Lebanon, so I decided to apply there.

I found my way to Canada where I declared my intention to apply as a political refugee. Following a three-week-long bureaucratic process, I was provisionally accepted as a political refugee. I stayed in Toronto with some distant relatives who were kind enough to guide me and help me find a place to stay while I continued the immigration process. There were numerous applications and immigration hearings, but after one year, I was ultimately denied refugee status. I was devastated—I didn't know where to go from there.

At twenty years old, Canada deported me back to the United States. They brought me back to the immigration office in Niagara Falls, and after a few hours there, they told me I was free to go. It was about ten o'clock at night, and I remember asking them, "Could you call me a cab, at least?"

I ended up staying with a friend in Los Angeles—someone I knew since childhood—until I could figure out my next step. I was supposed to return to Buffalo with an attorney for an immigration hearing, but the fear of deportation from the United States kept me from going, and ultimately, I skipped it. As a result, I became an undocumented immigrant for a few years. Luckily, I was able to obtain permanent legal residency through a lottery system and received my "green card" to remain in the United States.

The devastation of being rejected refugee status in Canada ultimately turned out to be a blessing in disguise, as I much preferred living in California to Toronto. I continued to work full-time to pay for my education and completed my undergraduate studies at the

University of California, Los Angeles. I then attended dental school at the University of Southern California, partly because of the dental trauma I had gone through as a child and a teenager. For as long as I can remember, I had always wanted to be a doctor. I had a burning desire to be of service to others, to have such a positive impact on people to change their lives for the better. I found I could accomplish this in dentistry, and specifically through orthodontics.

Initially, I had no plans to specialize. I had planned to become a general dentist so that any patient in need of dental treatment would be in good hands. However, as I went through various specialty rotations, I fell in love with orthodontics. It is an amazing area through which one can have a profound impact on someone else for the rest of his or her life, especially for a child, despite the fact that it is not quite disease prevention.

Orthodontics is a combination of science and art. It allows me to build personal connections and relationships with people because of the treatment time, which spans over a long period. I see my patients frequently—much more frequently than I would as a general dentist. These were only the initial aspects I enjoyed most about orthodontics, and over time, I knew I had found my niche—my calling.

What Sets Orthodontic Centers of California™ Apart

Our mission at Orthodontic Centers of California™ is "to improve lives, one smile at a time," and our vision is to "be the leading orthodontic practice in California." We do this by focusing on delivering the highest quality of orthodontic treatment within a friendly and relaxed environment, while maintaining a patient-centric experience.

We don't want anyone who visits our office to be left behind—we do not want anyone unable to afford treatment to leave without exploring their options for better health, whether it's physical (in the sense of their bite or alignment) or emotional (the appearance of their smile and how they feel about themselves).

In California, there is a government-funded program called Denti-Cal, which is essentially a dental version of California's Medicare. Most orthodontists in our area do not accept patients on Denti-Cal because of the low reimbursement rate, which is about 50 to 60 percent less than usual customary reasonable (UCR) fees. Unfortunately, the majority of such patients are children who lack the proper dental education to maintain good oral hygiene, and the resources for oral disease prevention and cure, much the same way I lacked the proper education and resources to maintain a healthy mouth when I was a child.

Many of these children have mixed dentition—some baby teeth and some adult teeth—and would benefit from early, interceptive orthodontic treatment (also known as Phase One treatment) to prevent further complications from developing in the future, especially during their adolescent and teenage years. There are very specific criteria I look for when deciding whether or not we should start Phase One treatment. This is basically a checklist of what to look for before making that decision, as my treatment philosophy is to make the choice that is always in the best interest of the patient. While those indications for Phase One treatment are somewhat technical, they include things such as severe skeletal discrepancies (where the jaws are not aligned properly), oral habits such as thumb sucking (which can cause problems such as open bites), severe crowding (overlapping of the teeth), and psycho-social reasons, such as the child being the victim of intense bullying from peers due to the appearance of their teeth and/or bite.

Many of my Denti-Cal patients are children of immigrants, whose parents hardly speak any English. At no fault to them, these kids are in an environment where there's a lack of education in oral health. That's why I've made a commitment to treat underprivileged children with orthodontics, because I understand where they're coming from. Great care and service starts with our staff.

Our Staff

Our staff is committed to serving our patients and continually strives to improve the patient experience in our practice. We work with leading coaches in the industry and train with one of the largest dental consulting and training companies in the world. We invest in our staff and educate our team on world-class customer service and patient experience. I personally attend seminars and workshops on service and customer interaction. We hold leadership retreats and seminars where the entire staff, and specifically our leadership team, is exposed to new and emerging ways to better treat our patients and provide the best care experience. We also have on-site trainings every quarter with certified trainers, and are committed to systematically investing in our team through trainings to position ourselves to deliver the highest quality of service and care to every single patient that comes to our office.

These trainings are not about dentistry or orthodontics—it's nothing technical and is not for the purpose of improving our clinical technique (that's what continuing education courses are for). These courses and trainings are about exceeding patient expectations in the

1   "Oral health: A window to your overall health," Adult Health, Mayo Clinic, last modified April 30, 2016, https://www.mayoclinic.org/healthy-lifestyle/adult-health/in-depth/dental/art-20047475.

office, on how to over-deliver in service value from the moment they walk through the door and onward.

We take our time with every patient, new or existing. This helps patients feel relaxed, attended to, and not rushed. We have game stations in the office, which is a real attraction to many of our younger patients, and when they're ready, we bring them to the treatment bay. My very well-trained staff can calm patients down just through taking the time and talking through their treatment. There are no surprises. We tell them what we're going to do, show them what it looks like, and then proceed. For instance, if we're fitting a patient with braces, we let them know how they work: gluing the little brackets onto their teeth, etc. We emphasize that everything we do is virtually pain-free.

My staff is also aligned by seven core values that drive the patient-centric model of our practice. Knowing these core values and living them every single day makes it so that our patients can feel relaxed, comfortable, and know they can expect world-class results.

- ## Integrity

  In our practice, we hold our staff to a high level of integrity, as we're dealing with people who are trusting us with their children's or their own teeth.

- ## Positive mental attitude

  We recognize that occasionally we come to work with issues in the back of our mind, whether it's family issues, financial issues, or something more. However, it is a policy to shake it off when we're in the office. Once we walk through the doors, it's not about us anymore; it's about our patients. We're not here contemplating our problems—for the eight hours we are serving our patients, we are escaping from our own lives and impacting others in a positive way. I expect the entire team to show this positive mental attitude and put on a performance face, because our patients deserve nothing less.

- ## *Dedicated to the patients' best interest*

  Every decision we make in our practice is in the best interest of the patient. For example, I do not use molar bands which are large rings placed on back teeth. Many orthodontists routinely place molar bands on the first and second molars. However, because it is more difficult to keep teeth with molar bands clean, they often contribute to tooth decay. I have seen time and again decay formed under molar bands and as such, I've decided to forego these bands and place braces on all molars instead, despite it being a more challenging process. Braces are more hygienic and comfortable than bands and pose less of a cavity threat. This is just one example of acting in the patient's best interest.

- ## *Passionate about service*

  I expect passion from each member of my staff. To reiterate, our work is about our patients. We must have compassion when serving, and if this mindset does not resonate with my staff, then we're not a good fit for each other. I believe that one should be passionate about their job—if the passion is lacking, it's best to move on.

- ***Over-deliver in service value.***

  In our practice, we believe in the principle of over-delivering. What we give our patients should always exceed what they pay us to do.

  Anytime we take a dollar from somebody, we always want to give more than a dollar in service value. If we do not succeed in doing so, I do not feel comfortable taking anybody's money.

- ***Working in harmony***

  If there is no harmony within a team, then we're not a team, we are individuals. This core value is a crucial part of practice culture, which is key. In order to fulfill any other core values, it is imperative to have synergy and work as a team.

- ***Contribution and growth***

  As part of my team, team members are encouraged to participate in community service programs, such as our very own Orthodontics from the Heart™ program as well as contribute to the growth of our practice by spreading the word about us. More importantly, I am vested in the personal and financial growth of each team member—from supporting educational endeavors to financial growth.

I believe that alignment within the practice keeps everyone functioning at a high level, and this, in turn, helps us treat our patients with the utmost positivity and care. Not many other orthodontic practices will spend a small fortune to continually train their staff on the quality and consistency of their customer service. Again, our primary focus is the patient, and how we can make every single one feel welcomed and cared for.

In addition to keeping my staff aligned, our practice also prides itself in keeping up to date with the latest advances in technology for orthodontics. We use digital radiography, cloud-based charting, digital scanning for Invisalign—everything is state-of-the-art, including the Damon braces system.

Damon Braces System

The Damon braces system is one of the most advanced self-ligating bracket systems. The term "self-ligating" refers to little doors on the brackets which open and close, making it easier to work the wire through. This system is much more efficient compared to traditional braces most patients are familiar with, as those braces utilize elastic ties to hold the wire inside the braces. The elastic ties create a lot of friction, analogous to a bungee cord tied between the wire and the brace. This makes it difficult for the wire to slide around the braces, requiring higher forces to be applied. In turn, these higher forces translate to a little more discomfort and a higher level of pain when the teeth are moving.

In my professional opinion, Damon braces not only cause lower levels of discomfort, but they also expand the range of capabilities of orthodontic treatment with lower friction systems. Traditional orthodontic techniques have also involved frequent removal of four teeth in order to make room within the jaw bones for the rest of the teeth to grow into alignment. This is primarily because there is too much friction between the braces and the wires in these traditional systems to get enough expansion without pushing the teeth into unfavorable positions. With lower friction systems like the Damon system, we can frequently create space and relieve crowding without having to remove any teeth.

I've been using Damon braces for well over a decade, and it's the primary system I use within my practice to treat patients with brackets. However, I also have many patients who are good candidates for Invisalign, which I have also been using for over a decade as well. Clear aligners, of which the Invisalign brand is the most popular, is a household name, even though I believe this appliance may not best suit every case. My goal is to educate my patients on all available options. By showing them pictures and x-rays of their particular case and allowing them to make an informed decision, we help them achieve excellent treatment results.

Orthodontics from the Heart™

I was introduced to a non-profit organization called "Dentistry from the Heart" several years ago, which helps organize a free day of dentistry whereby doctors and staff can participate by providing treatment and dental cleanings for those less fortunate. As orthodontics was not their area of focus, my team and I decided to create our very own, orthodontic version called "Orthodontics from the Heart™" to make a difference in our very own community.

Our purpose with Orthodontics from the Heart™ is to provide free orthodontic treatment to children from low-income families, broken homes and foster homes, who otherwise would have no means of getting this much-needed treatment. We compiled a list of patients who had been to our office and reached out to them with information about the program. In order to quality for our free treatment, we asked children to write us a letter telling us why they thought they should be selected for orthodontic treatment through our program, and how this would impact their lives.

We received an overwhelming response and an outpour of letters with very touching stories. I read them with my family and staff, and we handpicked twenty kids who we felt the treatment would impact the most. My entire staff and associate doctors were thrilled to volunteer for the day. We opened our office for a full day in March 2018 and fit braces and other appliances on our pro bono patients, which we will continue to treat until completion. In terms of dollar value, we gave away approximately $100,000 of orthodontics that day. It was a day filled with joy—specifically the joy of giving to the less fortunate and impacting lives by reshaping smiles! The "icing on the cake" was being featured on a local news channel in a segment called "making a difference." I am committed to making a difference by making Orthodontics from the Heart™ an annual event.

Aside from Orthodontics from the Heart™, we also donate to charitable causes, such as supporting and donating to local schools in our area, various churches/temples, sports teams, children's hospitals, Los Angeles, and the Society of Orphaned Armenians.

I hope to make Orthodontics from the Heart™ a program which will involve other colleagues seeking to help their communities through orthodontics as well, because there are countless children in need of treatment they cannot afford. We can change so many lives with just one day of selflessness a year.

It's Not Too Late to Fix Your Smile

If there's one thing for you to take away from this book, I hope it's that oral health matters, and it is essential to the wellness of your or your child's overall health. Poor dental hygiene can contribute to and/ or worsen a host of problems, including diabetes and cardiovascular disease. As an orthodontist, I straighten teeth and fix smiles—which, to many may not seem very critical to health, but it's critical to the self-esteem of a growing child amongst peers at school, or even to an adult trying to take the next step in his or her career. It's more than just orthodontic treatment; it's a step toward a better life.

I had full orthodontic treatment when I was thirty-four. I was in residency and knew how awful my bite and my teeth were from my younger years. One of my co-residents worked on my teeth and it made a significant impact on my life. There I was—a man in my thirties, no longer afraid to smile or to speak to people.

Again, a lot of people are not well informed when it comes to oral health and hygiene. Other than education, I can't think of much else besides orthodontics that a parent can spend hard-earned money on that's going to stay with their children for the rest of their lives; it is an investment with a guaranteed return.

Orthodontics may seem like a large financial commitment when you think of it as paying for treatment up front. However, if we consider the lasting positive impact it can have over a lifetime, then we see that we're investing money into a powerful gift that can change a life forever. Looking through this long-term lens, orthodontics isn't costly at all.

However, the practice of orthodontics is not identical. It is very important to have treatment done right the first time. I have seen countless cases of poor orthodontics since I started practicing over thirteen years ago. I take great pride in providing a high level of orthodontic treatment. I often get referrals or transfer patients who started treatment elsewhere and were very unhappy with their results or experience. Many doctors do not accept transfer patients, but I believe, "Someone needs to treat these kids or adults. Someone has to take over, because if they're trapped in an office where they're unhappy, then they will not have a way out."

I want to rest my head at night knowing I've done the best I can every single day to make sure my patients have the best care, treatment, and experience in my practice than anywhere else. I hope that as you read this book, you'll come to not only feel more comfortable speaking with your orthodontist about your treatment options, but be more aware of what a significant impact it can make on your or your child's life.

Chapter One

THE PATIENT-CENTRIC PHILOSOPHY

Tell me if this sounds familiar: You open the door to a medical office and the first thing you notice is the harsh smell of disinfectant. There are a bunch of old, worn out chairs lining the walls—none of which are comfortably facing the television screen that's displaying static—and stacks of outdated lifestyle magazines are scattered on the scarce side tables. And at the furthest end of the room is a sliding glass window, scratched and smudged with fingerprints. Behind them sits an assistant who somehow doesn't see you standing at said window for at least two or three minutes after you've arrived.

At some point, we came to accept this kind of treatment as the norm; that we weren't people as much as we were penitents, come to beg for a moment of time with the almighty Doctor, and even if we'd scheduled an appointment, we were willing to wait for hours—half our day, even—for what ultimately amounts to five minutes of attention.

This is not how it should be.

Five Reasons People Don't Like Doctor Visits

From the Huffington Post

1. The doctor doesn't listen
2. The long wait
3. The doctor doesn't care
4. The doctor makes too much money
5. My dog gets more respect

A large part of the dissatisfaction with doctor visits is created by the environment and the doctor's non-patient-centric approach to delivering treatment. Most people's perception of a medical office, in other words, is that sliding glass window, the clipboard of medical questions, and the long wait until you're beckoned behind the door and into a treatment room. From the moment patients step in the front door, they're treated like a piece of paperwork because in the end, that's really all they're seen as.

The Patient-Centric Model

Our office couldn't be further from this dated, frustrating approach. For one, we don't even *have* a sliding glass window.

Words that Describe a Patient-Centric Model

Comfortable

Relaxed

Understood

Important

Satisfied

Listened to

Cared for

Respected

The system we have created in our office is what's called the Patient Centric Model. The entire experience is crafted around putting the patient first, with predetermined steps that include speed when speed is necessary, clear communication, and treatment that is well above the norm.

Creating a Five-Star Experience

When you walk into our office, our focus is on getting you to where you need to be as fast as possible, streamlining paperwork so that there's time for true comfort and relaxation. To accomplish this, we extensively train our team on what both the patient and the doctor require so there are as few hiccups in the process as possible.

This attention to detail and process goes well beyond the evident. For instance:

- *Answering the phone right away*. This may seem obvious, but try calling your physician right now. If you're like most, your call was probably received by an automated answering service that made you pick a number, and then another number, and possibly even a third number, just so you can leave a message on an answering machine. This is not the case at our office. Our phones are answered quickly by a real person so that we can address your needs promptly.

- *Flexible Schedule*. We strive to keep flexibility in our schedule so that if the need occurs, we can see you quickly—if not the same day—at a time that's as convenient as possible.

- *Clean Spaces*. Every space associated with our office, from our parking area to the storage closet, is kept clean and in good condition. The common areas and restrooms are clean and comfortable, and lightly scented so that they don't smell medical while at the same time, not overpoweringly fragrant. And there's no such thing as a worn or dirty surface in our office space. We make it a point to keep all glass surfaces clean, the paint fresh, and the furniture in good, clean condition.

- *Reception Desk*. Gone are the days of the non-responsive front desk person behind a tiny sliding glass window. Not only have we removed the window, but the front desk is also open and uncluttered, with a smiling front desk operator that greets you the moment you walk up. There is no waiting for someone to get off the phone and, if you were able to fill out our online forms ahead of time (sent directly to your preferred email address), there's usually no clipboard, either.

- **Waiting Room**. The waiting room is not only clean and tidy, but it's also completely devoid of old, worn, and rumpled magazines. Instead, there's a wide variety of reading material for all ages, along with a comfortably placed television (on low volume with captions, on a non-news channel that isn't discussing medical or dental procedures), and free wi-fi. We also offer chilled bottled water, coffee and tea, along with other patient amenities.

- **Treatment Bays**. We understand that the fear factor for dental offices is real and pervasive in our society. For that reason, when you walk into a treatment bay, you're not going to see a lot of medical equipment sitting out. Instead, we use soft lighting, tasteful decorations, and comfortable furniture to create a more relaxed experience.

- **Our Appearance**. This may not seem like an obvious importance, but we have several rules regarding the appearance of staff and doctors in our office. Uniforms must fit correctly—neither too tight nor too loose—and doctors must wear dress clothes with a clean, white lab coat whenever necessary. Everyone, from the front desk to the doctor, must be well-groomed with tattoos covered and any body piercings removed. It may not seem like a lot, but a clean and tidy appearance—from the rooms to the staff and even the doctor—lets our clients know that we pay attention to detail, and that every detail gets professional treatment.

Perception Is Everything

A story I've often heard attributed to Don Burr, founder of the former People Express Airlines, does an excellent job of pointing out the importance of attention to every detail.

Picture yourself the last time you had to fly somewhere. Imagine you had a pretty ideal experience this time around—you checked in early online, the line for security was minimal, and your gate was conveniently close to a cafe with clean, available tables. When they called your flight, you got onboard without a hitch, found a spot for your luggage right over your seat, and got into your seat without stepping over two other people or ticking off the other passengers around you.

Everything was going brilliantly until you sat down and unfolded the tray table and there, on the surface of the table, was a huge, crusty food stain. In that moment, you suddenly became convinced that the pilot was incompetent, the wings were held on with duct tape and the engine was one decrepit shiver from bursting into flame.

> Perception is everything, and if we aren't paying attention to detail, then dentists can be rest assured that their clients *are*.

Everything about your visit, from the moment you arrive, should feel like a five-star experience.

A fair number of patient satisfaction surveys suggest that while patients may like their doctor, they are most dissatisfied with the treatment they received from supporting team members. This is why our focus is a complete 180 degrees from the typical medical office experience—we spend an enormous amount of energy and effort making sure that our team is always present and aware of our clients' needs. Our staff know—and agree—that their needs come second to the needs of our patients.

From the moment you walk in the door, your experience dictates your relationship with us. Creating the best first impression requires substantial energy and effort, but if the end result is that our clients feel more comfortable, less fearful, and more respected by our doctors and staff, then it's all worth it.

Category of One

What is a "category of one" dental practice?

It's an orthodontic practice that values the power of distinction versus the cost of blending in. It's one that goes above and beyond for its patients, creating an environment that's difficult—if not impossible—for others to duplicate.

This distinction doesn't just apply to our physical building, however. It's also found in how we treat our patients and in the services we provide. For our patients, we want to give them the kind of smile that doesn't just serve its purpose, but stands out. A "category of one" company is, at all times, a reflection of the utmost quality in all aspects of its operation and it's this type of practice that we aim to exemplify every day.

Chapter Two

WHAT IS AN UNHEALTHY SMILE COSTING YOU?

As humans go, our greatest fears are pretty specific: there's extinction, of course, as well as physical injury, loss of autonomy, separation, and ego-death.[1] If you were to put these in order, extinction would be the most powerful, followed by the others in this same order, ending in ego-death, which can also be described as "embarrassment, humiliation, or any other form of strong self-disapproval."

So, where does "fear of dentistry" fall in this? It depends on how you view a dentist visit. More than likely, it falls first under the fear of physical injury—that we'll somehow feel pain during our visit. This isn't

---

1   Karl Albrecht, "The (Only) 5 Fears We All Share," Psychology today, last modified March 22, 2012, https://www.psychologytoday.com/blog/brainsnacks/201203/the-only-5-fears-we-all-share

an uncommon fear. In fact, about 75 percent of all U.S. citizens have some degree of fear of the dentist, from mild to severe, with anywhere between 5 and 10 percent of the population experiencing true dental phobia, meaning that they'll avoid a dentist's office at all costs.[2]

What is that "cost," by the way? What is fear costing us when we won't go to the dentist because our gums bleed a little when we brush or because that one tooth is really starting to ache more often?

What are the opportunity costs of fear?

When we look back at things we've done in life that we were initially afraid of, we most often find that those fears were simply built up in our own head.

Take Geoff's story, for instance. At forty-one years old, he was only able to visit a dentist under IV sedation, and had been that way for at least twenty-five years. For Geoff, this severely limited the dentists he could go to, and meant that he only saw them when something was wrong. In this particular case, he arrived at a dental hospital with tooth pain and an examination showed that he had no less than three teeth that needed to come out. After he had them extracted under sedation, however, Geoff was able to undergo therapy that allowed him to slowly ease into a dental office and eventually have a tooth restored and two cavities filled with just a local anesthetic; with no IV and fully conscious.[3]

If Geoff had been able to deal with his fear earlier in life and simply visited his dentist regularly, it's likely he never would have needed such extensive work done. That is, in a nutshell, a whole bunch of opportu-

---

2   Peter Milgrom, Philip Weinstein, and Tracy Getz, *Treating Fearful Dental Patients: A Patient Management Handbook, 2nd Edition* (Seattle, WA: University of Washington, Cont, 1995)

3   K.I. Wilson and J.G. Davies, "A joint approach to treating dental phobics between community dental services and specialist psychotherapy services – a single case report," *British Dental Journal* 190, no. 8 (April 2001): 431–2, https://doi.org/10.1038/sj.bdj.4800993a

nity costs—by choosing to let fear keep him from the dentist, it cost him twenty-five years of proactive dental visits, tooth pain from lack of treatment, dental damage, and likely the impact to his self-esteem for a quarter of a century because of a poor smile.

When you think back on your own life, it's likely there are more than a few instances where you had to walk through your fear instead of backing away from it—and you probably found out that you'd made it a lot more frightening in your own head than it was in actuality.

Are Bad Teeth Telling Your Life Story?

Your smile tells your life story faster than any other means known to humanity. First impressions are made in milliseconds, and while research is still trying to pinpoint all the details of how we're able to assess people so quickly, we do know that common facial features play an incredible role in other people's initial—and lasting—perception of you.

"A first glance at a person's face often leaves a lasting impression," writes psychologist Vivian Diller in a July 2012 article for *Psychology Today*. "Facial features are more often remembered following initial interactions than people's bodies or even their personality traits."

Diller goes on to note several conclusions that people make based on their first impression of our eyes, nose, skin, and hair, as well as our smile and our teeth, all of which are viewed and assessed in less than a second.

"A person's smile is the feature that elicits the most immediate and positive reaction from others," Diller states. "People who have a spontaneous and natural smile … send an inviting message to others. It says 'come join me, talk to me.'" An unsmiling face, however, can say, 'I'm not interested.' A frown says, 'go away.'"

Teeth, too, leave a strong impression. "While we may not all have dazzling straight pearly whites, having good oral hygiene goes along with the positive impact that a great smile brings," writes Diller. "Severely crooked or yellowing teeth can imply you are a smoker or heavy drinker. Mottled teeth can reflect certain illnesses, poor nutrition, or an eating disorder. Fresh and bright teeth generally suggest that you are someone with a healthy lifestyle and good grooming habits."

Photogenic or Not, Good Teeth Matter

Good teeth are a hot topic on the acting website Backstage.com. In an article titled "Nothing But the Tooth," actors speak to how improvements to their smiles made significant differences in their careers.

"Before I got my teeth whitened, they [casting directors] made comments suggesting that I was not going to be on TV," said actress Sonora Chase. "That has changed."

Actress Jessica Delfino also shared that a quality veneer made all the difference in her performing career, taking her from being self-conscious about a poorly repaired front tooth to having the confidence to take on the "perfection-loving media."

According to Dr. Michelle Callahan, "Whether we like it or not, we are often judged by our appearance...your smile has more of an effect on what others perceive about you than you think."

In a perception study conducted by marketing research firm Kelton, more than a thousand participants were asked to give their honest opinion on the people in a variety of images, and what they found was that those with straight teeth appeared to have more desirable qualities than those with crooked teeth, including the snap judgment that they were "happy" and "professionally successful."

In comparison to people with crooked teeth, the perception study also noted that Americans perceive those with straight teeth as being:

- 45 percent more likely to get a job
- 58 percent more successful
- 57 percent more likely to get a date
- 47 percent more likely to be viewed as healthy

Additionally, close to three in five Americans would rather have a nice smile than clear skin, and 87 percent would give up something for a year if it meant having a nice smile for the rest of their life.

So what story is your smile telling others? And just as importantly, how is that story affecting your *life story* going forward?

"Research clearly shows that having decayed or missing teeth has a strong negative impact on self-esteem," notes psychologist Daniel W. McNeil, PhD. "It also has an impact on employability."[4]

Bad Teeth, No Job

When the American Dental Association took a look at oral health and well-being in the United States in 2015, it uncovered some

4   Rebecca A. Clay, "Drilling down on dental fears," *Monitor on Psychology* 47, no. 3 (March 2016): 60, http://www.apa.org/monitor/2016/03/dental-fears.aspx

alarming statistics. Young adults were almost neck-and-neck with low income adults in agreeing that "the appearance of my mouth and teeth affects my ability to interview for a job," and one in four adults avoid smiling due to the condition of their mouth and teeth. Judging by what we just learned from psychologist Vivian Diller, this means that a quarter of adults are unintentionally hurting the first impression they give others just because they're too embarrassed to smile.

For a case in point, just look at the story of "Shelly" as reported by the Deseret News in Salt Lake City, Utah.

In 2012, a counseling office in Salt Lake City was looking for a front desk employee and while they were getting plenty of applicants, none met all of their specific qualifications. Then, Shelly arrived at the office as a temp. A thirty-five-year-old mother of three, she was reportedly "pleasant to work with, competent, and kind to the patients." In fact, another front desk employee urged leadership to hire Shelly on permanently. Yet, when her temp position ended, the company chose not to bring her on.

When asked why Shelly wasn't hired, employees were apparently told that it was because she had bucked, crooked teeth.

"He [the office manager] said it wasn't the image we wanted to project at our clinic," said one of the front desk employees.[5]

Image is the New Communication

Communication is becoming more and more image-focused, with social media reflecting this through a massive uptick in video messaging. As of 2017, more than 70 percent of Gen-Z (those born after 1995) spent

---

5   Mercedes White, "No teeth means no job," Deseret News, last modified December 27, 2012, https://www.deseretnews.com/article/865569512/No-teeth-means-no-job-How-poor-oral-health-impacts-job-prospects.html

more than three hours a day watching videos online, and their social platforms of choice, such as SnapChat and Whisper, are almost solely image and video-based.[6]

While most employers aren't as obvious about their motivations in hiring or not hiring certain individuals, you can be certain that a good smile is going to play a big part in other people's first and ongoing impression of you: a factor that a woman in California was well aware of as she sat outside of a state dental clinic overnight.

At fifty-three years old, Patty knew she needed dental work if she was going to land a job. As she waited outside of the clinic, she told an NBC news reporter about her five broken teeth, three cavities and gum abscess, and how the pain was only part of the reason she was there—she knew the condition of her teeth was an important part of the hiring process.

"I really don't smile a lot," she told the reporter. "I know that when you have a job, you want to have a pleasant attitude and you've got to smile and be friendly."

The report went on to quote Dr. Susan Hyde, a dentist and population scientist at the University of California in San Francisco, "If you want to portray someone as being wicked, they have missing front teeth. If they're ignorant, they have buck teeth. Even from a very early age, we associate how one presents their oral health with all kinds of biases that reflect some of the social biases that we have."

Dr. Lindsey Robinson, dentist and president of the California Dental Association, added, "Customer service jobs, good entry-level

---

6   Nelson Granados, "Gen Z Media Consumption: It's A Lifestyle, Not Just Entertainment," Media & Entertainment, Forbes, last modified June 20, 2017, https://www.forbes.com/sites/nelsongranados/2017/06/20/gen-z-media-consumption-its-a-lifestyle-not-just-entertainment/

jobs ... they're not available to people who have lost the basic ability to smile, to function, to chew properly."[7]

But the chain of consequences resulting from bad teeth doesn't stop here. Poor dental health can also affect your immediate health, and apart from making it difficult to work when you're not feeling well, it can affect your long-term wellbeing and can even result in death.

A Heart Attack ... and Diabetes, Stroke, and Cardiovascular Disease ... Waiting to Happen

In 2007, a twelve-year-old boy in Washington, D.C. died from a toothache. It was a combination of unfortunate circumstances that led to the tragic event, but ultimately, what could have been an $80 routine extraction ended up costing him his life. His family paid close to $250,000 in medical care, including brain surgery in an attempt to save the boy from the infection that had spread from a tooth abscess into his brain.[8]

This is an extreme instance, but the fact is that bacteria, which accumulate quickly in the mouth as they feed on the food particles surrounding un-brushed teeth, have instant access to the blood-stream through the inflamed gums that occur with periodontal disease. These bacteria don't go through any filtering process, either, as they would if they entered the body through the lungs, stomach, ears or nose. In other words, inflammation, the gaps created by a

---

7   Jonel Aleccia, "Bad teeth, broken dreams: Lack of dental care keeps many out of jobs," NBC News, last modified June 12, 2013, https://www.nbcnews.com/feature/in-plain-sight/bad-teeth-broken-dreams-lack-dental-care-keeps-many-out-v18906511

8   Mary Otto, "For Want of a Dentist," Washington Post, last modified February 28, 2007, http://www.washingtonpost.com/wp-dyn/content/article/2007/02/27/AR2007022702116.html

receding gum line, and other untreated dental conditions, are akin to having an un-bandaged open wound on your body. Those bacteria can jump right in and start wreaking havoc, which is why researchers are discovering that there are more diseases than just the obvious ones associated with poor dental health.

The following links between poor dental health and disease are described in depth by the National Institute of Health's report "Oral Health in America: A Report of the Surgeon General": https://www. nidcr.nih.gov/DataStatistics/SurgeonGeneral/sgr/home.htm

- **COPD**. COPD, or chronic obstructive pulmonary disease, is caused by chronic bronchitis, emphysema, or recurring respiratory infection, and has been associated with periodontal disease due to bacterial pneumonia living in the mouth and making its way into the airway.

- **Diabetes**. Periodontitis has been linked to diabetes— both types 1 and 2—so often that it's now being referred to as one of the main complications of diabetes. Reports have suggested that it's a two-way street for these diseases, as well—that diabetics are more likely to get periodontal disease, and periodontal disease may have a negative impact on glycemic control.

- **Heart Disease and Stroke**. Evidence is continuing to grow on the relationship between infectious agents and systemic diseases, with certain bacteria that thrive in dental infections being identified as potentially linked to heart disease. For example, as we said earlier, bacteria or viruses in the mouth can get directly into the blood stream, where they can cause inflammation, blood clots, and narrowing of the arteries.

- **Preterm Birth and Low Birth Weight**. Bacterial infection in the mouth may contribute to adverse pregnancy outcomes, as the harmful bacteria and other toxins created by the infection can get into the blood, cross the placenta, and harm the fetus. Additionally, the reaction of the mother's immune system to the infection could directly or indirectly interfere with growth and/or delivery.

This Isn't Just About Teeth—It's About the Rest of Your Life

This book isn't about promoting dentistry. It's about helping you discover the long-term opportunity costs of fear and the importance of being proactive about the health of your smile.

The first step is understanding the importance of a healthy mouth, which you should have a better idea of after reading this book. The next step? Understanding that when you're not healthy, you're not living at your full potential.

Chapter Three

UNLEASHING HUMAN POTENTIAL THROUGH ORTHODONTIC TREATMENT

At the age of fourteen, Susan still remembers the conversation that took place between her dentist and her parents, when her dentist first urged them to take her to an orthodontist. There was some medical terminology batted about, but one line stuck with her so clearly that she can still hear her dentist saying it today; "If you don't do something now, we'll probably have to break her jaw when she's older."

If she hadn't heard her dentist say that, she might have fussed a little more about the braces her orthodontist fitted her with, but instead she took it all in stride and even switched out her bracket bands to reflect the holidays as they went by. A little over a year later, the braces came off and everyone in the office "ooh"ed and "ahh"ed over her beautiful smile.

Fast forward to a little over two decades later and thirty-seven-year-old Susan couldn't quite remember when she stopped wearing her retainer, though she was sure it was within a year or two after getting her braces off, and certainly before she went to college. Consequently, her teeth had drifted to the point where she could noticeably tell a difference in how they sat in her mouth.

One of the issues people face when it comes to maintaining a healthy smile is the lack of clarity around the natural aging process and its impact on your teeth. Orthodontic relapse is a condition that a lot of post-braces patients fall victim to, and one that we see in our orthodontic offices pretty frequently. The issue is that people rarely understand the importance of wearing a retainer and the fact that time and other dental conditions down the road can all affect the hard work that your doctors put into that straight smile so many years ago.

After braces, teeth need at least one year to stabilize and get used to their new positions in the jaw. This is when retainer wear is at its most important—to protect the teeth from relapsing into their former positions and allow them time to solidify in their new positions in the jaws. We suggest wearing retainers full-time during this one-year period. If a retainer isn't worn, or is worn infrequently, during this time, the teeth may shift and if the patient doesn't visit her dentist, she may not notice that shift for some time.

Even if a retainer is worn for at least a year, after the patient stops wearing it, the teeth once again fall victim to outside—and inside—influences. Teeth grinding, for instance, can place strain on the teeth of the upper jaw, and tooth loss can cause the remaining teeth to drift into the vacant spot. Internal influences could be genetics, which can prompt your teeth to shift, for instance, or gum disease can cause the structure to weaken. Our routine protocol is to wear retainers full-time for at least a year, every night for the following two years, and then gradually reduce to no less than two nights a week, indefinitely.

And then there's simply the age factor. As we age, pressures on the teeth can cause them to shift, so even if Susan did wear her retainer for a few years after braces, twenty years is a long time for teeth to react to any influences, internal or external.

In neglecting her teeth, Susan neglected the potential that straight teeth could have resulted in. Apart from generally giving her a healthier appearance, straight teeth also create a healthier mouth in actuality—with straight teeth, there are fewer places for food and bacteria to hide, making it easier to brush. And straight teeth also make chewing easier, which means less strain on the jaw, which means avoiding jaw joint issues down the road.

It's like the old adage "for want of a nail, the kingdom was lost." By not maintaining a healthy smile and being proactive about it, we open the gates to numerous problems down the road. For Susan, drifting teeth meant that they were sitting in less-than-ideal positions in her mouth, making them harder to brush, which meant more bacterial buildup. And more bacterial buildup can cause inflammation of the gums. Inflammation leads to gingivitis, gingivitis leads to periodontal disease and periodontal disease leads to … well, you read the last chapter, right? It could potentially lead to anything from heart disease to death.

All for the want of proactive, preventative dental care.

Hitting the Reset Button On Your Smile

Unlike many things in life, you have the option of hitting the reset button on your smile. It doesn't matter if you've smoked your whole life or if illegal drug use has caused most of your teeth to rot out—whatever you've done, technology and advancements in dental science have made it possible to rebuild just about any smile.

We live in a world today where photos are uploaded by the billions every single day. In 2014, for instance, it was estimated that every two minutes, the same number of photos were uploaded to the Internet as existed in the world one hundred and fifty years ago. This is a world where you can no longer hide your smile.[9] The camera is on you constantly and whether or not you realize it, it's having an impact on the course of your life. People make snap judgments based on the images they see of you, and based on their first 0.1 seconds of interacting with you. You're regularly being assessed in situations and under circumstances where you cannot speak for yourself—your image is doing all of the talking.

I'm aware this probably sounds superficial, but regardless of our better efforts, we're still a superficial species. Our instincts still react the same way they did eons ago—an attractive smile still triggers the selection of a mate. It still inclines us to like or trust someone more. Genuine smiles, also called Duchenne smiles—the ones that get you to use those little muscles around your eyes—also signal to others

---

9   Rose Eveleth, "How Many Photographs of You Are Out There In The World?" The Atlantic, last modified November 2, 2015, https://www.theatlantic.com/technology/archive/2015/11/how-many-photographs-of-you-are-out-there-in-the-world/413389/

that you're focusing on just them, which in turn encourages them to cooperate with you.[10]

At the same time, the way you feel about your smile also influences your own perception of self. Your self-concept is determined, many times, by the way you look at yourself in the mirror. Do you smile at yourself from ear to ear or do you frown in an effort to conceal your imperfect grin? That perception lives with you and reflects outward, whether you realize it or not, affecting not only your own happiness, but the happiness you could be generating in others.

There is no doubt that a bright and vibrant smile can do more to drive happiness in someone's life than you would think on the surface. When you think about it, what are the things you could do in life that will ultimately drive happiness? Most likely, the majority of those things can be traced back to your ability to smile.

What Makes Us Happy?

Research shows that around 40 percent of our own happiness is under our control. So what can you do to make yourself happier - and how do those behaviors relate to your smile?

---

10   Gil Greengross, "Want to Increase Trust in Others? Just Smile," Psychology Today, last modified April 30, 2015, https://www.psychologytoday.com/blog/humor-sapiens/201504/want-increase-trust-in-others-just-smile-0

1. Strong relationships with people you trust
2. Good income / paying bills without stress
3. Taking the time to think about the good things in life
4. Performing voluntary acts of kindness
5. Exercising
6. Living life instead of buying things
7. Living in the moment - mindful meditation
8. Time with friends

Unleashing Human Potential

A lot of people ask me what I do professionally, and when I tell them that I'm an orthodontist, the typical reaction is, "Oh, you straighten teeth, right?"

If only it were that simple.

One of the big reasons I got into orthodontics was because I realized the power that a confident smile can give someone. And I realized that when people have a smile they can be proud of, they show it a lot more.

I found that the more people smiled, the more confident they were and the easier it was for them to speak and communicate. These people had a higher self-image, and a better self-concept. And believe it or not, I found that the more people smiled, the more career and professional success they experienced and the more productive relationships they had.

So when people jump straight to "you straighten teeth" once I tell them I'm an orthodontist—well, it's not nearly that simple.

What I and everyone else in our office are in the business of doing is unleashing human potential. We help our patients regain their ability to smile, and by doing so, we also help them acquire confidence, capability, and allow them to be more ready to take on the opportunities in the world and achieve great success for themselves and for their families in the process.

Case Study: What Yearbook Smiles Tells Us

Over the course of thirty years, Drs. LeeAnne Harker and Dacher Keltner followed the lives of one hundred women after graduating from college to determine if a positive emotional expression in their yearbook photo was linked to their life outcomes.

During the study, Harker and Keltner, along with their research team, contacted the women in the study at ages twenty-one, twenty-seven, forty-three, and fifty-two, asking them various questions about marriage, family, and work, among other topics. What they found was that "over time, women who expressed more positive emotion in their yearbook pictures became more organized, mentally focused, and achievement oriented, and less susceptible to repeated and prolonged experiences of negative affect." In addition, they confirmed theories that "individual differences in positive emotional expression were linked to personal stability and development across adulthood, the impressions and reactions from other people, and the marital satisfaction and well-being up to thirty years later, "adding that, "People photograph each other with casual and remarkable frequency, usually unaware that each snapshot may capture as much about the future as it does the passing emotions of the moment."[11]

Overcoming Fear with Practice

Now that you understand the fear, the consequences, and the motivation of a healthy mouth, let me share with you how we're working to change the dental and orthodontic experience forever. The first and most important step is education—knowing the *why* behind a timely visit to the orthodontist—but the next is on me and my team, which is to make those visits the absolute best they can possibly be. Doctors can't afford to continue with the old-fashioned model of making patients wait on them. Today, it's the complete opposite. Only those doctors that are willing to put their patients front and center—to cater to *their* needs instead of the other way around—are the ones that are going to survive. And we intend to do more than survive—we intend to make your needs our number one priority, and in doing so, become *your* number one orthodontist.

---

11   LeeAnne Harker and Dacher Keltner, "Expressions of Positive Emotion in Women's College Yearbook Pictures and Their Relationship to Personality and Life Outcomes Across Adulthood," *Journal of Personality and Social Psychology* 80, no. 1 (January 2001): 112–124, https://doi.org/10.1037/0022-3514.80.1.112

Chapter Four

BEST TEAM IN TOWN

Over the years, I've spent a lot of time developing clinical skills, attending advanced training courses and doing everything I could think of to offer my patients the best and most up-to-date care possible. What I was missing, however, was the understanding that my team is the most impactful reflection of my ability. I could go through all the training in the world, but if lackadaisical staff members are treating my patients poorly, that knowledge and experience would never counterbalance that negative first impression.

Today, I understand that we have to stay at the highest possible level of clinical skills, training, and technology, not only to keep up with the rapidly evolving pace of dental technology, but to also provide our patients with the absolute highest quality of service.

The "best team in town" concept is our belief that we should not only have the most competent clinical team on the floor, but also a team that is present in all situations and circumstances, has been trained to stay focused on the patient, and a team that will never compromise on their work. This means that everything from the way appointments are scheduled when you call to how you're greeted when you walk in the door, how you're escorted to the treatment bay, and even how you are communicated with should be top-notch and focused only on you.

It's Not a Job, It's a Career

One of our primary goals is to turn each role at our office into a career. This means reinforcing each team member's overall commitment to the practice and the patient, connecting them to the mission of our organization and encouraging them to apply our core values both personally and professionally.

Our Core Values

1. Integrity
2. Positive mental attitude
3. Dedicated to patients' best interest
4. Passionate about service
5. Over-deliver in service value
6. Working in harmony
7. Contribution and growth

Through modeling core values, it's our hope that our staff will have more of a positive impact simply through the behaviors they exhibit, particularly when interacting with patients and with each other.

In other areas, we strive to make a positive impact by providing our staff with the best training, coached in the understanding that we expect from them the highest level of commitment and expectation. As a patient, we want you to understand that we're taking all of these steps to dramatically improve your experience. Our training both in clinical skills and continuing education are not just a "bare minimum" effort, but are undertaken in order to stay ahead of the curve and at the top of our game.

One of these efforts ties directly into our desire to be a Patient-Centric office, which is engendering in our staff—and particularly our team of clinical assistants—the desire to not just treat the patient, but to be their Oral Health Advocate.

Consider the following feedback we received from a hygienist shortly after going through patient-centric training:

The Honest Truth: *A Statement from a Veteran Hygienist*

The biggest problem that I see with other hygienists in other offices is that they aren't stepping up to the plate to be their patients' Oral Healthcare Advocate … not just a hygienist. I'm not pointing fingers—I've been in those shoes.

I used to tell a patient what they needed to know about a procedure, and when they showed the slightest pushback, I would give up. I didn't know how to handle their irritation, their impatience, and their questions about financing, but I realized that was my fault. And because I didn't know how to communicate how big of an impact this decision was going to have on their life, they didn't get the care that they deserved.

As hygienists, if we don't step up for the patient, then we are the ones that are keeping a problem alive that has existed in the dental industry for way too long.

I still remember the day that this was made real to me. I was standing in the break room, drinking coffee and complaining about the training session that I and the other staff members had to take that day. We walked into the training room, all of us still highly skeptical. But then, the trainer started talking, and the truth of what she said hit me in the stomach. How she described the importance of advocating for our patients changed the way I looked at my career forever. From that day on, I knew I couldn't keep doing things the same way. I was no longer an "oral janitor" but an Oral Healthcare Advocate. My life's purpose is to give my patients healthier smiles and healthier lives, and to get as many other people to join me as possible. I'm telling you, I'm ready to start a revolution.

What I do is not just a nine-to-five job. It's not just a paycheck. Being a hygienist is our chance to serve—and to save lives. During my training, I realized that, as Oral Healthcare Advocates, we're literally the only people in our patient's lives that are aware of their oral health, so we can't be afraid to tell them what they need to do. Our patients trust us 100 percent to tell them what treatment is the best possible one for them.

As a hygienist, if you know that a procedure will benefit your patient, but you don't give 100 percent effort in educating them on it, then you are doing that patient a serious disservice. They don't know what you do, but they want to understand and they won't know what to ask unless you give them as much information as you can.

That's just the honest truth. If you're doing any less, then you aren't fulfilling your duties as a healthcare provider. It isn't that you have bad intentions if you don't—none of us do! Since becoming a hygienist, I've realized that the people in this industry are some of the warmest, most caring individuals I've ever met. But this epidemic of apathy has to stop. Some hygienists are out there doing the bare minimum of service rather than consistently over-delivering to their patients—being reactive instead of proactive about their treatment. I know that we can do better than that.

During training, our team learned to refocus on what each patient truly needs, and we made it our mission to give him or her the best solution. I now feel empowered to give my patients a healthier life and to take responsibility for that patient like I would a member of my own family.

Continuing Education

In addition to standard and continuing education, our staff may be participating in upward of one hundred hours of training per year on subjects directly related to the customer experience, such as the oral healthcare advocate training the hygienist spoke to earlier.

Our focus is on having a consistent process for everything from the front desk to the treatment coordinators, to clinical assistants, to the doctors in the practice. It's these processes that allow us to work with the other professionals in our office so that every patient receives the same, consistent quality of care.

Our Office is a "No Judgment" Zone

Let's address the elephant in the room right now—people judge. They judge us by our appearance, by the clothes we wear, by our opinions, even by the way we cut our hair. That may be able to slip under the radar at other establishments, but that attitude of judgment is left at the door at our office. If any one of our employees walks in with a judgmental chip on their shoulder, then that's the day they lose their job.

We do *not* judge anyone who comes to us. We do not allow any unchecked personal opinions from our team members drive how you are treated. We don't treat you differently based on what type of insurance you have or if you don't have insurance—we're simply interested in understanding what it is you need or want to have done, making sure you're comfortable, and providing you with what you need.

As a doctor, we want our patients to understand that this is not a normal commitment, but it is one that I believe is key to the relationship we share with our patients and the reason why our number one source for new patients today is referrals from existing ones.

Chapter   Five

STEWARD OF YOUR SMILE

Let me ask you a question—have you ever worn down your tires and gotten a flat?

If so, what did you do? Did you go to the mechanic and ask for a patch, or did you get a new tire?

A lot of us have opted for the patch—even when the tires are so worn they're practically bald because we tell ourselves that we just can't afford new tires right then. When that happens, however, what do we end up doing? Eventually we have to get that new tire, but we're spending more for it because we've had to pay for the patch and any other damage that happened to the car from running on bald tires until we bought new ones.

More often than not, we do more damage and end up costing ourselves more when we choose to "patch" instead of truly repair.

It's the very same situation with your smile. Your teeth bear much of the brunt of your lifestyle. If you enjoy acidic beverages such as coffee, wine or energy drinks, then that enamel is getting worn down every day. If your diet is high in sugar, then your teeth are constantly being bombarded by bacteria, and that's even if you're brushing the recommended two times a day (which a staggering one in five people *do not* do).

Taking care of your mouth is more than just brushing—there's a lot more that goes into it, and yet so few of us are on the preventative side of smile care. For instance, tell me—do your gums bleed when you brush? Do you ever notice a little bit of a gap between your gum and your tooth when you feel around your teeth with your tongue? Or is there buildup on a tooth or two that you just can't get off with brushing?

All of these conditions—gingivitis, receding gum line, and plaque buildup, respectively—are signs you need to see your dentist as soon as possible, and yet so many of us ignore these kinds of issues until they start to hurt. And by then, the conditions have likely progressed to point where more involved treatments may be necessary.

It's the strangest thing! We could go see the dentist every six months, get our teeth cleaned, floss regularly, and let the dentist take care of minor cavities as they occur, or we could do as more than a third of Americans do and just not go to the dentist until those preventative conditions become a severe problem.[12]

Acidic and sugary drinks and snacks aren't the only challenges that our teeth face on a regular basis. There's also the impact of stress on teeth—grinding (also called "bruxism") is associated with anxiety

---

12   Lecia Bushak, "Oral Health Isn't Much Of Americans' Concern, Poll Finds: One-Third Didn't See The Dentist Last Year," Medical Daily, last modified April 29, 2014, http://www.medicaldaily.com/oral-health-isnt-much-americans-concern-poll-finds-one-third-didnt-see-dentist-last-year-279468

and depression, and can cause you to wear away your enamel and expose the dentin, which is much softer than the enamel and can lead to sensitivity and cavities.[13] It could even cause your teeth to crack and, over the long-term, it can lead to complications with your jaw joint (also called the "TMJ" or temporomandibular joint) and may even cause facial muscles to become enlarged from overuse, potentially blocking your salivary glands, which then can lead to inflammation, pain, and dry mouth … which leads to more cavities, and so on.[14]

We define stewardship as "protecting and growing the owner's assets with fierce intensity." Therefore, taking stewardship of your smile is about recognizing that your health is a valuable belonging, and taking those preventative measures is paramount to maintaining your oral health so you never reach the point of paying $10,000 for a repair that could have been a minor fix if you'd seen your dentist on a regular basis.

When you do run into those repairs, though, stewardship is also about making the best choice for your smile rather than the cheapest one. Remember the tires analogy? Patching your problem ultimately ends up costing you more than getting it right the first time. And as your orthodontist, I never want to encourage you to just patch something five or six times when we can eliminate the problem once and for all.

---

13   Angelina R. Sutin et al., "Teeth grinding: Is Emotional Stability related to bruxism?" *Journal of Research in Personality 44*, no. 3 (June 2010): 402–405, https://doi.org/10.1016/j.jrp.2010.03.006

14   Donna Pleis, "Teeth Clenching And Grinding Can Affect Your Dental Health," Bruxism, Colgate, last modified, http://www.colgate.com/en/us/oc/oral-health/conditions/bruxism/article/teeth-clenching-and-grinding-can-affect-your-dental-health-1114

Why We Don't Care Who Your Insurance Carrier Is

When it comes to your health and your smile, my first thought is always going to be "What's the right thing to do here?" It's about what we can do to protect you and help you grow and live a full and happy life. If a close relative comes to me with a dental condition, for instance, I'm not going to tell her how to patch it for now—I'm going to tell her how to fix it for the long-term. And the same goes with my patients—I don't want to recommend temporary repair when you will be far better served in the long-term by fixing it right the first time.

This is why we don't care who your insurance carrier is. Ultimately, your insurance is never going to give you everything you need. We accept it, but if it costs more, then we'll find a way to make it work. Financing is readily available and there are ways to make it affordable. But insurance should never be the deciding factor. We are taking care of *you and your family*, not your checkbook, and how well you take care of your mouth impacts every aspect of your life from the day you're born and will follow you to the grave.

What Is the Cost of Neglecting Your Dental Health?

Health is an interesting value. It's something we all need and yet, it's not something we can purchase. We can't walk into a gym and say, "Okay, I'll take two well-defined biceps, a washboard stomach and a set of toned glutes. How much will that be?" Instead, we have to work hard to produce and maintain a healthy body on our own.

It takes time and it takes discipline, but for the sake of our overall health, it's worth it.

When we say "worth it," however, what do we mean? There's the personal, innate worth, of course—the cost of time and effort put into brushing our teeth or hitting the gym are "worth" it when it leaves us feeling healthier. But there are also physical financial benefits to good health, as well.

One economics researcher, Michael Grossman put it well when he described human behavior regarding health: "Individuals inherit an initial stock of health that … can be increased by investment," adding that "Individuals 'choose' their length of life" when investments are made through direct inputs into that stock, such as medical care, diet, exercise, and recreation.

If you really enjoy reading into the process of creating economic models, then you should certainly check out Grossman's paper "On the Concept of Health Capital and the Demand for Health." Otherwise, I'll just get right to one of his conclusions, which is that when we take stock of our life (or, in this case, look at it like investing in stock), we can predict that the more educated people are about the benefits of good health, including longevity, the more proactive they'll be about obtaining it.[15]

Consider the following study conducted by a group in Scotland, who set out to determine whether or not a country-wide nursery tooth brushing program was not only making a difference in the longer term dental health of children, but if it was also saving money on dental costs down the road. Specifically, the study looked at the cost savings from improvements in the dental health of five year olds

---

15   Michael Grossman, "On the Concept of Health Capital and the Demand for
       Health," *Journal of Political Economy* 80, no. 2 (April 1972): 223–255, https://
       doi.org/10.1086/259880

through the avoidance of needing extractions, fillings, or other treatments due to decay.

The first step was determining the complete costs for filling or extracting a decayed primary tooth, and then on average, how many of those dental treatments were conducted over a ten-year period.

They found that not only did the dental treatments for five year olds decrease over time once the tooth brushing program was initiated, but by the program's eighth year, the expected financial savings alone were two and a half times the cost of the program.[16]

How, then, can we be proactive about dental health? With two simple initial investments:

1. Brushing and flossing at least twice a day

2. Visiting your dentist at least twice a year.

That's all the investment you need to make on a stock that can have incredibly rewarding returns.

Opportunity Costs of Dental Health

Essentially, an opportunity cost is the choice that you give up when you make a decision. That is, when given the choice between "gum" and "a mint" and you choose "a mint," the opportunity cost is the gum.

When you expand on that idea, "opportunity cost" not only stands for the loss of one choice in preference of another, it also represents the long-term consequences of your choice.

If we stick with the gum/mint choice, for instance, by choosing the mint, we could, say, miss out on the longer-term benefit of

---

16 Yulia Anopa et al., "Improving Child Oral Health: Cost Analysis of a National Nursery Toothbrushing Programme," *PLoS ONE* 10, no. 8 (August 2015), http://doi.org/10.1371/journal.pone.0136211

chewing gum. If the gum was sugarless and the mint was not, we'd be taking a hit on calorie intake by choosing the mint (as well as doing just that much more potential damage to the teeth thanks to that extended sugar exposure). Extrapolate that even further and maybe chewing gum could have kept us from thinking about eating a snack—but by taking the mint, we experienced a sugar spike and now we're eating a burrito at 2:30 p.m. instead of taking a walk, and by the end of the week, we've gained three pounds.

Opportunity Cost of Dental Health

OPTIONS:	*brush and floss teeth everyday*	*OR*	*don't brush and floss teeth everyday*

CHOICE: *don't brush and floss teeth everyday*

WHY? *because I don't have time*

COST: *new implants to replace the rotten ones*
$3,000 to $6,000 per tooth

Opportunity costs can be subjective, but they can also be quite objective and practical. In this case, consider the opportunity cost of deciding not to brush and floss every day.

The mouth is the perfect breeding ground for bacteria, and not just one type, either—there are close to four hundred different species of microorganisms, mostly bacteria, living on every filmy surface and in every hard-to-brush crevice.

According to dental researcher Sigmund Socransky, "In a clean mouth, one thousand to one hundred thousand bacteria live on each tooth surface. A person who doesn't have a terribly clean mouth can have 100 million to one billion bacteria growing on each tooth."[17]

While a good amount of those bacteria and microorganisms are beneficial, helping to fight off disease-carrying microorganisms that try to enter the body through the mouth, the oral cavity can also house harmful bacteria that, if not brushed away, can eventually irritate the gums, causing gingivitis, which evolves into periodontal disease. At this point, some of the most direct results of poor dental health may occur, including bad breath (otherwise known as halitosis) and tooth loss.

I discussed several of the following related conditions in an earlier chapter, but they're important enough to bring up again as the stewardship of your dental health can quite literally mean the difference between life and death. Those open, bleeding gums provide instant access to the bloodstream, where their presence has been linked to conditions such as:

- **Dementia**: researchers following more than five thousand people for eighteen years found that those "who reported not brushing their teeth daily had a 22 percent to 65 percent greater risk of dementia than those who brushed three times a day." Another, smaller study on Alzheimer's has noted that the brains of those with the disease exhibited more bacteria associated with gum disease than those without the mental illness.

- **Endocarditis**: bacterial infection of the lining of the heart and its valves, causing inflammation and infection

---

17   Jane E. Stevens, "Oral Ecology," MIT Technology Review, last modified January 1, 1997, https://www.technologyreview.com/s/400012/oral-ecology/

- **Heart disease**: wherein harmful bacteria make their way directly to the heart

- **Stroke**: bacteria-related inflammation of arterial walls and blood clotting can cause the arteries to narrow and lead to stroke

- **Rheumatoid arthritis**: periodontal disease can increase the pain caused by this disease

- **Lung disease**: both pneumonia and chronic obstructive pulmonary disorder (COPD) can be worsened by harmful bacteria making its way from the mouth to the lungs

- **Brain Abscess**: as noted earlier in the case of the twelve-year-old who died from a decayed tooth-related brain abscess, bacterial infections of the mouth can be life-threatening if left untreated. [18]

It only takes about three days of not brushing for detrimental conditions to form. Once you pass seventy-two hours, the volume of bacteria will have reached the point where they're producing enough acid to carve holes in tooth enamel, and plaque may have solidified to the point where it becomes difficult, if not impossible, to remove without professional intervention.[19]

What, then, is the opportunity cost of choosing not to brush and floss your teeth at least twice a day? It could be the cost of a filling, an implant, dentures, your overall health and even, your life.

---

18   Lauren F. Friedman, "13 Awful Things That Happen If You Don't Brush And Floss Your Teeth," Business Insider, last modified February 14, 2014, http://www.businessinsider.com/what-happens-if-you-dont-brush-and-floss-your-teeth-2014-2

19   Jane E. Stevens, "Oral Ecology," MIT Technology Review, last modified January 1, 1997, https://www.technologyreview.com/s/400012/oral-ecology/

Steward of your Smile

In our office, we adhere to the stewardship model, which is to protect you, to help you make good decisions and to help you grow as a person through the things that we can have an impact on.

When it comes to treatment, first and foremost, we believe in being good stewards of our patients, their time, their financial resources, and all of the transactions that occur in our business, which means helping our patients steward over their decisions in a meaningful and productive way. This is because we've found that many non-patient-centric offices will guide their treatment path based upon what they think the ability of the patient is to pay. This is simply *not* the philosophy that we use.

Instead, we treat you as a person and make recommendations to you as though you're a member of our family and allow you to ultimately make the decision that's right for you. We believe in providing you with the best recommendation for your condition, and the only way to do that is to leave the question of funding out of the picture.

As I pointed out earlier, there are times when budgets require people to patch something, be it a leak in a pipe, a hole in a weak roof, or a tire. But when we think about that decision over the long run, patching is pretty much a guaranteed way to have the problem return, and likely in a worse way than the first time around. This is why we like to give patients the option to fix things correctly the first time since it winds up being more cost effective and better for the patient overall.

Take the leaking pipe, for example. Patched, it may work a little while longer, but when it starts to leak again, that leak will likely go unchecked for a certain period of time and eventually cause more damage than it did when it was patched. The cost then ends up being the cost of fixing the problem correctly and repairing the damage done in the meantime. So which is the more cost-effective solution?

Convenient Financial Arrangements

When we consider the financial part of any visit to our office, we always approach it with these words in mind: flexible and without fear. We don't want to avoid discussing it—it's something we'll need to talk about anyway, so why not get it out there? But we don't want it to be awkward or to become a barrier to working with us. For these reasons, we offer multiple options for patient financing, including flexible, interest-free payment plans.

In all cases, we like to provide our patients with options because there are times when we need to patch, but we always make sure to provide all of the information for the appropriate fix, as well, and discuss financial options if the budget is a problem. Above all, it's important to us that we educate our patients on the conditions resulting from either decision, including the consequences of patching versus fixing something correctly. Ultimately, the choice is in the patient's hands inside of our practice.

Chapter Six

THE POWER OF A FREE DAY OF ORTHODONTICS

One of the foundations of our practice is financial stewardship, and an important part of that is committing to living off of less than you earn, and giving a portion of what we make to the community. We do this through several means, but one of the means where we feel we make the most impact is in our annual day of free orthodontics, wherein we provide free orthodontic treatment to members of the community who need it. The day is called "Orthodontics from the Heart™", modeled after a similar program called "Dentistry from the Heart", and it's not just our doctors providing voluntary services, but our entire team as we lend our skills to help those who need it most. This mentality of giving back is a part of our culture and one we're more than happy to nurture. It reminds us of how fortunate we are to do what we do, to work with the people we work with, and to be able to give, with our time, our knowledge, and our resources.

Dentistry from the Heart

Dentistry from the Heart began as a single event in the Tampa suburb of New Port Richey, Florida, in early 2001. The brainchild of Dr. Vincent Monticciolo, the intent of that first event was to provide relief to the many bay area residents that were in desperate need of dental care. The concept—which remains the same to this day—is to provide a free extraction, filling or cleaning to whoever needs it, no questions asked.

Being an exclusively orthodontic practice, we have modified the program and called it Orthodontics from the Heart™, where we spend the day starting free orthodontic treatment on members of our communities that cannot afford it otherwise. We continue treating them over the following two or three years, until completion of their treatment.

"Most patients opt for the extraction," said Michelle Sotil, director for Dentistry from the Heart. "Usually because they're dealing with some form of untreated dental disease or another condition that requires immediate attention."

The day of the first event, Dr. Monticciolo pulled up to his office to find a line around the block, with some having stood there since the night before in order to be first in line for the free services. The event was so successful that other practices throughout Florida began picking it up and from there, the event has spread to dental practices throughout the world.

As of 2018, there were more than three hundred Dentistry from the Heart events held in the United States each year, as well as in Canada, Ireland, New Zealand, Australia, and Puerto Rico.

"It's truly a wonderful charity, and each year it gets bigger," said Ms. Sotil.

While Dentistry from the Heart is a one-day event, participants in need of additional care are typically given information on nearby dental schools and free clinics for follow up treatment.[20]

The Impact of a Free Day of Orthodontics

Steven was the sixteenth person waiting in line for a Orthodontics from the Heart™ day. He was twenty-five years old and for the past five months, he'd been suffering from pain on the right side of his lower jaw. When we finally got him in a chair, the infection was so bad that extraction was really the only option.

Although no one is ever happy to lose a tooth, Steven was grateful for the service, stating that if it wasn't for the free day of dentistry, he wouldn't have been able to afford to have the tooth removed as he'd lost his job months ago and was having trouble finding work. In fact, a cousin of his went to the emergency room for a tooth infection a few months back, only to learn that the ER wasn't equipped to handle dental issues, which is the case with most emergency rooms across the country.

Low Income Adults and Poor Dental Health

According to a report by the American Dental Association's Health Policy Institute, of the low income adults surveyed:

---

20 Jody, "Dentistry From The Heart: From Day-of-Care Event to International Dental Nonprofit," Dentistry From The Heart, last modified August 10, 2017, http://dentistryfromtheheart.org/blog/director-of-dentistry-from-the-heart-michelle-sotil/

- 35 percent are embarrassed about the condition of their mouth and teeth
- 42 percent have difficulty biting and chewing
- 29 percent believe that the appearance of their mouth affects their ability to interview for a job
- 74 percent accept that they'll lose teeth with age, compared to 48 percent of high income adults
- Pain is the number one oral health problem suffered[21]

Unfortunately, this story isn't unusual. According to the American Dental Association, (ADA) "most hospitals don't have the facilities or staff to provide comprehensive dental care. So many patients receive only antibiotics or pain medication, but the underlying dental problem is not addressed. In too many cases, the patient returns to the emergency room with the same problem—or worse."[22]

Emergency room visits for dental pain have increased significantly over the years, with 2.1 million visits in 2010. Most of these were for non-traumatic dental conditions, and a 2015 ADA report estimates that up to 79 percent of dental-related ER visits could have been diverted to dental offices.[23]

---

21 "Oral Health and Well-Being in the United States," American Dental Association's Health Policy Institute, last modified 2015, http://www.ada.org/~/media/ADA/Science%20and%20Research/HPI/OralHealthWell-Being-StateFacts/US-Oral-Health-Well-Being.pdf?la=en

22 "From the Emergency Room to the Dental Chair," American Dental Association, http://www.ada.org/en/public-programs/action-for-dental-health/er-referral

23 Thomas Wall, Kamyar Nasseh, and Marko Vujicic, "Majority of Dental-Related Emergency Department Visits Lack Urgency and Can Be Diverted to Dental Offices," American Dental Association's Health Policy Institute, August 2014, http://www.ada.org/~/media/ADA/Science%20and%20Research/HPI/Files/HPIBrief_0814_1.ashx

Preventable Dental Emergencies

Dental ER visits doubled from
1.1 million in 2000 to 2.2 million in 2012

2000   2012

ER visits cost 3 times as much
as dental visits

dental visit   ER visit

80% of dental-related ER visits
are due to preventable conditions

Up to 1.65 million ER visits can be
referred to dental clinics

Source: American Dental Association, ADA.org

What the ADA goes on to point out is that an increasing number of adults are forgoing regular dental care for a number of reasons, including the fact that dental benefits coverage has continued to decline for working-age adults.[24]

"The problem, while worse among lower income brackets, affects people across the economic spectrum," the ADA states, which is just one reason why programs such as Orthodontics from the Heart™ are becoming increasingly important.[25]

24   Thomas Wall and Marko Vujicic, "Emergency Department Use for Dental Conditions Continues to Increase," American Dental Association's Health Policy Institute, April 2015, http://www.ada.org/~/media/ADA/Science%20and%20Research/HPI/Files/HPIBrief_0415_2.pdf?la=en

25   "From the Emergency Room to the Dental Chair," American Dental Association, http://www.ada.org/en/public-programs/action-for-dental-health/er-referral

How We Participate

In 2018, Dentistry from the Heart founder Dr. Monticciolo provided care to more than five hundred people at his New Port Richey clinic. At our practice, we strive to help as many people as we can during our free day of orthodontics event, which is held in December before the holidays.

For more information on when our next free day of dentistry event takes place, please visit our website www.OCCSmiles.com.

Chapter Seven

BEGIN WITH THE END IN MIND

Did you know that between the ages of twenty and sixty-four, adults average about seven lost permanent teeth? And about 10 percent of Americans between the ages of fifty and sixty-four have *no* teeth left?[26] That's a lot of tooth loss, and if you're thinking right now that this average loss is probably greater on the older adult end than the younger adult, consider the following statistics from the American Dental Association's Health Policy Institute:

- Young adults are the most likely to report problems due to the condition of their teeth and mouth.

---

26   Lauren F. Friedman, "13 Awful Things That Happen If You Don't Brush And Floss Your Teeth," Business Insider, last modified February 14, 2014, http://www.businessinsider.com/what-happens-if-you-dont-brush-and-floss-your-teeth-2014-2

- 35 percent of young adults have difficulty biting and chewing

- 33 percent of young adults avoid smiling due to the condition of their mouth and teeth

What was also surprising about that report was that only 37 percent of the adults participating in the national survey reported that they'd visited the dentist in the last year, and only 77 percent planned to visit one in the coming year. This, despite the fact that just about all of them (95 percent) agreed that regular dental visits keep them healthy and a majority (82 percent) believed that a straight, bright smile will help you get ahead in life.[27]

Okay, enough statistics. What it comes down to is that dental health is incredibly important at every age, and at every stage in your life, you risk dental health issues. As we age, the risk rises, which is why it's our job to remind you that the decisions you make about your dental health today are going to stay with you for the rest of your life. If you neglect your teeth now, chances are that you'll need more work later down the road and if you neglect those bigger repairs, then you might end up being one of those ten-percenters without any teeth whatsoever.

Coming back to the importance of good stewardship, not only is it beneficial to see your dentist regularly, but it's also important to know the kinds of dental conditions that you can expect with age as your teeth wear, and as any work you've had done begins to break down and your gums begin to recede.

---

27 "Oral Health and Well-being in the United States: Data & Methods," American Dental Association's Health Policy Institute, 2015, http://www.ada.org/~/media/ADA/Science%20and%20Research/HPI/OralHealthWell-Being-StateFacts/Oral-Health-Well-Being-Methods.pdf?la=en

For instance, I've been shocked to have people come in that undoubtedly need orthodontic treatment, for reasons other than just for aesthetic improvements, and yet they tell me they don't feel like treatment is necessary. But if you think about the long-term benefits of straight teeth and a correct bite as described previously, not treating the condition could lead to further breakdown of teeth and the potential increase in the rate of cavity formation, and much more complex and invasive treatment in the future.

We don't want this or any procedure to be a surprise to you. Instead, it is our job to teach you about the natural progression of dental care and at what stages you may expect to take some extra preventative steps to keep your mouth healthy over the long term.

You can eliminate a lot of pain, discomfort, and frequent visits to the dentist by being proactive about your dental health. Our goal is to educate you so that you never feel that we're trying to "get" you to do something you don't want to do.

Check out the chart on page 71. There, you can jump to the most common dental conditions that are occurring at your age. I would suggest that you read it so you can have a good understanding behind any of the suggestions we make to you the next time you visit our offices. If you choose not to take preventative measures, that's your decision to make. However, know that if you choose to neglect your teeth for long periods of time, then you should budget to fix your teeth and take care of any related health conditions that may arise because of that neglect.

The best way to think about this is to begin with the end in mind. As you near the end of your life, what kind of teeth do you want to have? If you're like most people, then what you want is to have real teeth and a real smile. And you can have that—if you first understand that it is your responsibility to achieve it. As doctors, we're simply your partner and a provider of solutions to help you achieve your goals. It's on you to take the actions necessary to make those goals happen.

Part Two

Your Mouth at Every Age

Dental Expectations at Every Age

Childhood

Ages 0-6

Teaching proper toothbrushing

Treating common dental emergencies

- Knocked out tooth
- Cracked tooth
- Tongue or lip bite
- Toothaches
- Objects stuck in teeth

Fluoride treatment

Ages 7-9

First orthodontic visit

Establishing proper eating habits—avoiding sugary drinks and foods

Applying dental sealant (painted on child's 1st & 2nd molars as they emerge)

Pre-Teens and Teenagers

Reinforcing proper eating habits

Greater likelihood of cavities

Hormonal impact on oral health

Ages 20-39

Increased risk for gingivitis

Risk of TMJ pain due to:

- Tooth movement or other dental conditions
- Injury
- Craniofacial muscle spasms
- Rheumatic disease
- Other factors that cause the temporomandibular joint to shift

Stress impacts on oral health

- Tooth grinding
- Cracked teeth

Maintaining orthodontic adjustments (such as wearing a retainer after braces)

Ages 40-59

Increased risk of periodontal disease

Maintaining annual comprehensive periodontal evaluation

Old cavities may have to be crowned, or the tooth removed/replaced

Increased risk of obstructive sleep apnea

Maintaining preventative dental care

Ages 60+

Risk of cavities and tooth loss increases

Risk of gum recession

Risk of dry mouth

Reapplying fluoride varnish

Dental implants and dentures

Impact of osteoporosis on oral health

Watching out for signs of oral cancer

Dental care and dementia

Dental concerns may seem to come up completely out of the blue, but more often than not, they've been around for a while—we either just didn't notice them before or chose to ignore them until the irritation or pain become too much to bear. That's one of the biggest problems with dental issues—you could have a cavity and not even realize it until it becomes so deep that it hits the nerve. Or you may have gingivitis and ignore that tinge of blood when you're brushing or flossing until it becomes a full on case of periodontal disease.

This is what is sometimes called the "treadmill of dental life." Decisions regarding your dental health can come at you so quickly that you have to make decisions that you don't want to make—such as extraction or surgery—because of the condition you're in. However, if you're consciously taking preventative actions on the front end, then that treadmill slows down and you either don't have to make those decisions, or you have a lot more time to consider your options because you're aware of the condition long before it becomes a serious issue.

In this section of the book, we'll look at many of the dental concerns that can occur over a lifetime and what you can be doing now to prevent them. Or, if you haven't taken preventative measures for some time (such as brushing regularly and seeing your dentist at least once a year), this section should give you an idea of what conditions to expect at your current life stage.

For more information, or if you'd like to book an appointment, please call us at (833)-OCCSmiles or email us at info@OCCSmiles.com.

Chapter Eight

CHILDHOOD

Everyone has a childhood memory of what their first dental visit was like, which is why parents today are looking to make that experience better. They want their kids to look forward to seeing the dentist, which is why one of the first things we tell new parents is to take their children to the dentist by the age of one.

That may seem a little young, but think of this way: when babies are born, their mouths are sterile. Within hours, however, they're colonized with organisms that will stay with them for the rest of their life. These bacteria, protozoa, viruses, and yeasts are mostly harmless, but once they settle in, they start building a habitat that's more welcoming to other, less-harmless organisms. Once a baby cuts those first teeth, the bacteria that's most likely linked to tooth decay—*streptococcus mutans*—is also likely to make an appearance.[28]

One of our biggest concerns when a baby's teeth first start to come in is that of Baby Bottle Tooth Decay, also known as "bottle rot." This condition typically affects the upper front teeth and is caused by prolonged exposure to sugar-containing drinks—including milk (milk contains 12 grams of naturally occurring sugar per cup, otherwise known as lactose). Prolonged exposure can occur when a child is put to bed with a bottle, or if they use a bottle as a pacifier, and that sugar is the best way to activate the rapid growth of *streptococcus mutans.*

When sugar is present, *S. Mutans* feeds on it, releasing acids that can eventually eat away at tooth enamel, making room for plaque to grab ahold, which bacteria latch onto and from there, begin forming new holes. The more sugar that's added, the more this condition spreads until the mouth's natural cleanser—saliva—can no longer wash it away.

Even though a child will eventually lose his or her baby teeth, these first teeth play a very important role in life. They are needed for developing clear speech, chewing, and will also help the adult teeth come in correctly.

---

28   Jane E. Stevens, "Oral Ecology," MIT Technology Review, last modified January 1, 1997, https://www.technologyreview.com/s/400012/oral-ecology/

Toothbrushing and Dental Health Care for Ages 0–6

Infants

- For babies whose teeth have not emerged yet, use a clean, damp pad or washcloth to wipe your child's gums after each feeding.

- Only place formula, milk, or breast milk in bottles. Do not fill them with juice, sugar water, or soft drinks.

- Do not put an infant to sleep with a bottle. Bottles should be finished before nap time and bedtime.

- If an infant uses a pacifier, only give them a clean one—do not dip it in honey or other sugar-containing liquids.

1–3 years old

- When your child's teeth come in, use a child-size toothbrush and no more than a pinch (about the size of a grain of rice) of children's toothpaste to brush their teeth until three years of age.

- Encourage drinking from a cup

- Encourage healthy eating habits

3–7 years old

- Brush your child's teeth with a child's toothbrush and a pea-sized amount of children's toothpaste.

- If your child wishes to brush his or her own teeth, make sure to supervise the process to ensure that all of the teeth are brushed and all of the toothpaste is spit out instead of swallowed. Supervision should occur until the child is between the ages of six and seven.[29]

Dealing with Common Dental Emergencies

As many times as you've warned your child not to climb on top of the monkey bars, or open containers with his teeth, or ride his bike too fast (I could go on, but if you're a parent, you know what I mean), dental emergencies still occur. Here are a few ways to deal with them when they come up:

- **Knocked-out tooth**: try to put the tooth back in its socket without touching the root. If you can't, then either place the tooth in your child's cheek next to the gum, or if you're worried about the child swallowing the tooth, place it in a glass of milk. Then call your dentist immediately.

- **Cracked tooth**: rinse the mouth with warm water to clean it out and give the child a cold compress to place against the side of the mouth to keep any swelling down. Then call your dentist immediately.

- **Tongue or lip bite**: rinse the mouth with warm water and apply a cool or cold compress to the affected area.

- **Toothaches**: rinse the mouth with warm water and gently use dental floss to remove any food caught between teeth, as this can be exacerbating the pain. Call your dentist as soon as it is convenient.

- **Objects stuck in the teeth**: try to use floss to gently remove it, but if that does not work, call the dentist. Do not try to

---

29   "Baby Bottle Tooth Decay," Mouth Healthy, American Dental Association, http://www.mouthhealthy.org/en/az-topics/b/baby-bottle-tooth-decay

use a sharp, solid instrument to remove the object as it may cause further damage.

"Colorado Brown Stain" and the Introduction of Fluoride

You've probably heard about the importance of using toothpaste containing fluoride at every age, including those first toothbrushing years. There are a lot of reasons behind this, first and foremost that, while fluoride is added to tap water, very few people drink tap water anymore, opting instead for bottled water or filtered water (note, however, that "activated carbon" filters do not remove fluoride. Only processes such as reverse osmosis and deionization can remove the mineral).

Secondly, bottled water can be incredibly acidic. A study published in the Journal of Dental Hygiene found that, of the fourteen commercial bottled water brands tested, ten were acidic, with a pH of less than 7.

"Dental professionals continually educate patients on the dangers of consuming acidic food and drink due to their potential to contribute to dental erosion and tooth decay," the study noted, "However, water is not typically categorized as acidic." In investigating the pH values as reported on each of the bottled water manufacturers' websites, the researchers also found that the actual values were lower (more acidic) than those reported.

So why is fluoride added to water?

The discovery of fluoride and its dental benefits ironically began with the problems that fluoride was causing. In 1901, a young dentist named Frederick McKay arrived in Colorado Springs, Colorado, with the intention of opening a dental practice. What he found when he arrived was astonishing—the residents of the town had dark brown stains on their teeth, some so significant that "sometimes entire teeth were splotched the color of chocolate candy." Eventually, the condition became known as Colorado Brown Stain.

Apart from the coloration, however, the staining didn't seem to be causing any harm, and in fact, after years of research, McKay found that these mottled teeth were very resistant to cavity formation. Additionally, he found that city residents whose permanent teeth came in and calcified before the stains set in did not develop the stains later, so the staining had to occur while the teeth were developing.

It was later discovered that incredibly high levels of fluoride in the water were causing the brown stain—a condition that became known as "fluorosis." But lower levels of fluoride didn't stain and actually appeared to be beneficial. Later on, studies confirmed that fluoride ions easily absorb into the surface of teeth where demineralization has occurred, and bond with the enamel. The bonded fluoride then attracts other minerals, such as calcium, to the damaged area, thereby strengthening the tooth overall.

The next question to answer, then, was how the benefits of fluoride could be used without triggering the ugly staining caused by fluorosis. Decades after the cause of fluorosis was discovered, Dr. H. Trendley Dean, head of the Dental Hygiene Unit at the National Health Institute, began to study exactly how much fluoride needed to be in water before fluorosis occurred, and whether or not physically and cosmetically safe levels of fluoride in water would help fight tooth decay.

In 1945, Dean worked out a deal with Grand Rapids, Michigan, to safely fluoridate the town's drinking water over a fifteen-year period. After eleven years, Dean was able to confirm that children born in Grand Rapids after the fluoride was introduced were 60 percent less likely to develop cavities.

Today, fluoridation projects benefit more than 200 million Americans and fluoride can be found in just about every toothpaste brand on the market.

___

Ages 7–9: First Orthodontic Visit

The best time for a child's first orthodontic visit is between the ages of seven and nine. This may seem like an odd time since most children still have quite a few of their baby teeth at this age, but this is actually the perfect age to have a preliminary screening done to ensure that there are no issues developing, such as crossbites, over-, or under-bites.

If there is an issue, this age is also the ideal time to start Phase One Treatment, which focuses less on the teeth and more on changing jaw growth. The younger a child is, the easier it is to guide the jaw into a stable, ideal bite. Imagine how much more growth a seven year old has ahead of him or her, rather than a twelve or thirteen-year-old. When potential issues are caught during this window of opportunity, orthodontists can get a jump on corrections and reduce the amount of time that child will need to spend in braces later on.

Ages 6–12: Dental Sealant

Dental sealants are thin coatings painted on a child's first and second molars (which emerge around the ages of six and age twelve, respectively) that fill in the deep grooves of the tooth to prevent cavities. According to the Center for Disease Control (CDC), "once applied, sealants protect against 80 percent of cavities for two years and continue to protect against 50 percent of cavities for up to four years." This is particularly important as the permanent back teeth are where nine out of every ten cavities occur.

---

*Top Three Tooth-Rotting Beverages**

Sports Drinks

Sweetened Iced Tea Drinks

Energy Drinks

*People always say "Don't drink soda because of the sugar" but the truth of the matter is that a sugar-free energy drink is worse for your teeth than a classic cola, because it's more acidic. It's that combination of sugar and acid that does the most damage, but acid is ultimately worse on your teeth than sugar.

Chapter Nine

PRE-TEENS AND TEENAGERS

The pre-teen years are when you really reinforce the importance of brushing teeth twice a day on their own. At this point, your child should have already had their first orthodontist visit and may or may not be undergoing treatment to prevent a bite condition. Of all the things you can do for your child's dental health at this age, having sealants applied is one of the most important, if only for the long-term impact that this pretty simple process can have.

Eating for a Healthy Mouth

When it comes to maintaining overall mouth health, diet and nutrition are just as important as good brushing habits. Diet (the food we eat) and nutrition (the nutrients in the food) both impact the health of our mouth differently. Diet has a local effect, impacting the integrity of our teeth, saliva, and the mouth's pH balance, while nutrition has more of a systemic effect, impacting the integrity of the jaw bone, teeth, and supporting structure of the teeth. That is, changing your diet will more directly affect your mouth health while changes in nutrition will also have an impact, but it will happen over a longer period of time and affect the greater structure of the mouth.

Where we often run into trouble is the overconsumption of what's called "fermentable carbohydrates," which are those added and naturally occurring sugars in food. The difference between fermentable carbohydrates and other carbohydrates is that the fermentable kind breaks down in the mouth instead of later on in the digestive tract, sticking around to feed bacteria and launch the decay process.

Fermentable carbohydrates come in obvious and not-so-obvious forms. There are those foods that definitely contain sugar, such as candies, cakes, cookies, sodas, and chocolates. And then there are the less-obvious: bread, breakfast cereal, bananas, crackers, potato chips, pretzels and even dried fruit.

Additionally, the "stickier" these fermentable carbs are, the worse they are for your mouth, as they latch on to the nooks and crannies of the tooth and feed the bacteria that produces the acid that eats away at tooth enamel. "Sticky" doesn't just mean gooey and gummy in the way raisins and licorice are sticky—it can also mean "gets stuck easily" in the way potato chip crumbs can become wedged between your teeth and stick around long after you've finished eating them.

What are the best foods to eat for a wholesome diet, good nutrition, and an overall healthy mouth? The Dietary Guidelines created by the U.S. Department of Agriculture and the Department of Health and Human Services is a great place to start:

A healthy eating pattern **includes**:

- A variety of dark green, red, and orange vegetables
- Legumes (peas and beans)
- Grains, at least half of which are whole (brown rice, oatmeal, whole wheat bread)
- Fresh, whole fruits
- Low-fat or fat-free dairy, including milk, cheese, yogurt
- Protein foods, including seafood, poultry, eggs, lean meat, nuts, seeds, and soy products

A healthy eating pattern **limits** saturated fats, trans fats, added sugars and sodium, and includes consuming:

- Less than 10 percent of daily calories from added sugars
- Less than 10 percent of daily calories from saturated fats
- Less than 2,300 mg of sodium per day

If alcohol is consumed by adults of legal drinking age, it should be limited to one drink per day for women, and two drinks per day for men.

Every diet should begin with a strong base of grains as well as a daily intake of:

- 2 1/2 cups of vegetables
- 2 cups of fresh fruit
- 3 cups of calcium-containing milk, yogurt, and/or cheese
- Proteins (meats, beans, eggs, nuts)

And when it comes to snacking, try to choose non-sticky, non-fermentable carbohydrates. For example:

Best choice:

- Cheese
- Protein (meats, beans, eggs, nuts)
- Milk products (no sugar added)
- Water

Okay choice:

- Whole fruits such as apples and pears (these contain natural sugars, but have enough water in them that the sugar is diluted and saliva can more easily wash them out of the mouth)
- Vegetables (while vegetables contain carbs, they don't have enough to be dangerous)
- Unsweetened carbonated waters (these often contain a small amount of sodium)

Worst choice:

- Candy

- Cookies
- Crackers
- Bread
- Muffins
- Potato chips
- Pretzels
- Dried fruit
- Bananas
- French fries
- Cakes
- Soft drinks and other drinks containing sugar, including fruit juices

---

Ages 13–19: Treating Cavities

When lunch consists of a trip to the convenience store for a soda and a candy bar, cavities are eventually going to be an issue. A lot of teenage boys are full on into not taking care of themselves, and while girls tend to do a better job of taking care of themselves and their dental health, cavities can still become an issue—particularly if you have a family history of dental conditions.

Even though kids should already be seeing their dentist twice a year, this age range is when a bi-yearly checkup becomes incredibly important. Cavities need to be caught early and treated before they lead to further tooth decay.

When it comes to fillings, preference in the United States has more or less shifted away from silver amalgam and toward composite fillings, though there are a number of filling options available, and the procedure itself is pretty simple.

Types of Fillings

Depending on your preferences, the extent of tooth decay, and whether or not you have any allergies to certain materials such as metals, there are a number of options for filling materials, including:

- **Gold**: While expensive, gum tissues actually tolerate gold incredibly well and the fillings can last in excess of twenty years. However, apart from the cost, gold fillings also take longer as they often have to be made to order by a third-party lab before they can be cemented into place. This can require multiple visits before the procedure is complete.

- **Silver (amalgam)**: Also a material that's pretty resistant to wear, silver fillings also tolerate the heat and moisture of the mouth well, are relatively inexpensive, and last an average of fifteen years. However, since they're dark in color, they're more noticeable. Compositionally, most silver fillings are composed of mercury, silver, tin, copper, and other trace metals.

- **Composite**: This is increasingly the most used filling type as the color is much closer to the natural color of the tooth. However, they tend not to last as long as metal fillings, with an average lifespan of three to ten years depending on care, and common liquids such as coffee and tea can cause them to stain.

"Composite" is short for "composite resins," which is usually a combination of specialized plastics and a filler such as silica.

- **Porcelain**: Like gold, porcelain inlays typically need to be custom created by a lab and then bonded to the tooth. These fillings can be matched to the exact color of the tooth and can last between fifteen and thirty years. By nature, porcelain is also resistant to staining. These fillings, however, can be cost-prohibitive, with prices similar to the cost of gold fillings.

Basic Filling Procedure

1. The process of cleaning and filling a cavity begins with local anesthesia, which is used to numb the area around the tooth so that you don't feel pain during the process.

2. Then the decay is cleaned out using a small drill and shape the space so the filling will fit in tightly. If it's a bonded filling, the tooth will also get etched with an acid gel before placing the filling.

3. Finally, the filling gets placed on the tooth and polished to ensure that the filling is smooth and comfortable.

Cavities By Age

How likely are you to need dental care as you age? Check out these statistics from the United States National Health and Nutrition Examination Survey (1999 - 2004) on the percentage of adults in each age range with either a cavity, or missing or filled permanent teeth:

Ages 20–34: 85.58 percent

Ages 35–49: 94.30 percent

Ages 50–64: 95.62 percent

How Puberty (Hormones) Can Affect Your Teeth

Along with all the other changes your body goes through during puberty, one of the more overlooked ones is the change that happens with your gums.

Between the ages of eleven and thirteen, when puberty is most likely to occur, gum tissue becomes more responsive to the accumulation of dental plaque and may bleed and become inflamed more frequently. When these symptoms become more prevalent, the condition is generally referred to as chronic marginal gingivitis, or puberty gingivitis, and it's generally believed to be caused by the increased hormone levels that occur with puberty*.

Both males and females are susceptible to the condition, and its onset is believed to be predictive of the formation of more significant periodontal diseases later in life.

This is just another reason why good dental health is incredibly important in the pre-teen and teenage years, as proper oral hygiene today can be the difference between healthy teeth and gums for a lifetime.

*Of note, the hormonal changes that can occur with pregnancy and menopause have also been associated with an increased risk of gingivitis and periodontal disease.

Chapter Ten

AGES 20–39

The college years are another span of life where cavities are more likely to appear. The typical college diet doesn't help, with late-night study snacks coming into play more often and the general neglect of leafy green vegetables in one's diet. College is also when gum disease starts to pop up, starting out with the light bleeding of the gums during brushing, which is caused by gingivitis. If left untreated, those irritated, inflamed gums can quickly evolve into full on periodontal disease.

The good news is that gingivitis is pretty reversible during this age range. If you can get back into regular dental visits, regular cleanings, and brushing your teeth at least twice a day, the inflammation can go away without any permanent damage. If, however, the gingivitis goes for too long untreated, then not only will your teeth need to be cleaned, but your gums, as well, which is a much bigger deal. Think of it as similar to the condition that your car would be in if you didn't wash it for five or six years. You can't just drive that kind of buildup through the car wash and expect it all to come off—you have to get some serious detail work done.

What are the signs of gingivitis?

That little bit of blood in your toothpaste every time you spit? That's not supposed to be there. Gingivitis is the swelling and irritation of the gingiva, which is the part of your gum at the base of your teeth, and if it's not taken care of quickly it can lead to tooth loss, periodontitis, and other serious gum diseases.

Apart from a bit of blood when you brush, other signs and symptoms of gingivitis include:

- Puffy, swollen gums

- Dark red gums

- Tender gums

- Bad breath

- Receding gumline[30]

Gingivitis begins most often with poor dental health. When the biofilm on teeth isn't brushed away regularly, it can build up to form plaque, and that plaque is what causes irritation. Then, as the plaque builds, it turns into calculus—otherwise known as tartar—which is much more difficult to remove than plaque and is a breeding ground for bacteria. Only a professional dental cleaning can remove calculus. If that calculus isn't addressed, it will begin to irritate the gingiva,

---

30   "Gingivitis," Mayo Clinic, https://www.mayoclinic.org/diseases-conditions/gingivitis/symptoms-causes/syc-20354453

causing irritation, which then allows the gums to bleed more easily. This bleeding then opens the door to more bacteria getting directly into the gums and the bloodstream, leading to tooth loss, periodontitis and the risk of those diseases we mentioned earlier.

What increases the risk of gingivitis?

Poor brushing habits are the most common risk factor for gingivitis, but other conditions can contribute to the risk, including:

- Dry mouth

- Poor nutrition

- Dental restorations that don't fit well

- Crooked teeth that aren't cleaned well

- Conditions that cause a decrease in immunity such as HIV/AIDS, leukemia, or cancer treatment

- Smoking or chewing tobacco

- Old age

- Hormonal changes

- Genetics

- Viral and fungal infections

Headaches or TMJ Pain?

Of all of the hinging points in your body, the temporomandibular joint (TMJ, commonly called the "jaw joint") works harder than any other. Also, due to the combination of sliding motions and hinging, the TMJ is also the most complicated joint in the body. The jaw joint is where all of the major movements of your skull are centered and it is constantly moving, whether you're aware of it or not. On a conscious level, its active when we chew, speak, or yawn, and on a subconscious level its constantly making micro movements such as clenching, grinding, shifting, and repeatedly opening and closing.

Due to its connection to the trigeminal nerve—the largest of the twelve cranial nerves which run throughout the upper and lower jaws and into the teeth, eyes, and even the tongue—the smallest misalignment can have a significant impact on the rest of the system.

There are numerous conditions that may lead to TMJ pain, many of which become more prevalent as we age. These include:

- **Tooth movement or dental conditions** – tooth movement as we age, the wearing down of teeth, and tooth replacement, as well as dental procedures that change how our teeth interact, can affect the TMJ

- **Injury** – trauma to the jaw joint, head, or neck can have long-term effects that may not be felt until months or possibly years after the initial injury occurred

- **Craniofacial muscle spasms** – caused by injury or medications

- **Rheumatic disease** – this condition, which refers to a larger group of conditions that cause inflammation, pain, and stiffness of the joints, such as arthritis, can affect the TMJ as a secondary condition.

Common signs of TMJ issues:

- Facial aches and pains
- Frequent headaches
- Tooth wear

- Numerous dental problems (broken teeth, crowns or history of several root canals)
- Aches and pains around the ear
- Tender or painful jaw
- Discomfort or difficulty chewing
- Popping, clicking or grinding noise in jaw joints
- Difficulty opening and closing mouth due to locking of jaw joint

A significant sports injury in your teenage years or early twenties, or a car accident that seemed to only result in a case of whiplash, may evolve into issues with the TMJ later in life as the damaged jaw joints deteriorate under the tension of the unbalanced system.

What causes TMJ Pain?

Any time your bite changes, it affects your TMJ, and anytime your TMJ shifts, it can put mechanical stress on your teeth. Think of it like a finely tuned engine—if anything becomes misaligned, however slight, it will put stress on the system. As the stress increases over time, the misalignment becomes worse until the whole system becomes noticeably and painfully out of alignment.

Patterns of dental problems on the back teeth in particular can be a sign of undiagnosed TMJ issues. These problems can include root canals, missing back teeth, cracked teeth, broken porcelain fillings, etc., any of which can indicate that the system is under more stress than it should be. Additionally, teeth that are under additional stress from excessive bite force are also more likely to suffer periodontal problems.

One of the biggest problems with TMJ issues is how long they take to manifest. If headaches due to an injury that affected the TMJ don't appear until years after the incident, then it's not likely that the person suffering from them is going to make that connection.

Good dentists should be on the lookout for these types of conditions. If the alignment of the patient's jaw seems off, even if it's just slight, and we suspect a TMJ issue, then the first thing we'll do is test the diagnosis. This typically involves the patient being fitted with a type of mouth guard called an occlusal splint, which sets the jaw joint back into an ideal bite when worn.

An occlusal splint may look like a standard mouth guard, but it does more than just protect the teeth from grinding together at night. Instead, it is custom designed to hold the jaw in just the right position so that the teeth are aligned, relieving the muscle stress being placed on the TMJ by the misalignment.

After a few days of wearing the splint, the patient will come back in and we'll discuss the impacts, if any. If the patient is feeling forty or fifty percent better just from wearing it, then we know we're headed in the right direction. If they still feel the same and the headaches aren't getting any better, then we'll continue to fix the tooth issues that they originally came in to see us about and we'll likely refer that patient to another doctor. While TMJ issues are an often looked-over source of headaches and facial pain, other causes include ear infections, facial neuralgias (nerve-related facial pain), and sinus problems.

If the occlusal splint *is* making a difference, then the patient may wear it for anywhere from a couple of months to a couple of years until the jaw settles back into proper alignment.

Home Care for TMJ Issues

If you suspect that you have TMJ issues, there are some steps you can take at home to relieve the discomfort:

- Ice packs applied to the side of the face, particularly just in front of the ear where the TMJ is located

- Make conscious efforts to keep your face relaxed with lips together and teeth apart

- Eat softer foods

- Take small bites and chew with both sides of the mouth

- Don't rest your chin in your hand

- Don't bite hard objects, such as pencils, fingernails, cuticles, etc.

- Don't hold phones between the neck and shoulder

- Avoid excessive or extensive movements of the jaw, such as big yawns or chewing gum.

- Practice stress-relieving techniques

- Do gentle jaw stretches or jaw massages. One approach is to place your thumb or fingertip in the small "notch" located about one inch in front of your ears and on the underside of the cheekbone. Gently pressing inward and upward in this spot and rubbing in soft circular motions may provide some relief.

If the TMJ pain continues, there are other options for treatment, though each should only be considered after assessing all of the pros, cons, and risks with your doctor:

- **Pain medication:** muscle relaxers, pain killers and other medications as prescribed may help with the temporary relief of TMJ pain.

- **Dental adjustments:** this involves making changes to the teeth to bring the bite back into balance.

- **Botox**: Since Botox works by blocking the nerve signals to the muscles, it may provide temporary relief to sore jaw muscles when used in small doses, although this method is not approved by the FDA for use with TMJ issues.

- **Surgery**: While surgery is an option, it should be avoided where possible as there are no long-term clinical trials showing the effectiveness of surgical procedures helping with TMJ disorders, and the treatment is often irreversible.

- **Implants**: Artificial implants to replace jaw joints are also an option, but should also be taken under the same strict considerations as surgery.

For more information on discussions around TMJ treatments, visit the National Institute of Dental and Craniofacial Research's page on TMJ disorders: https://www.nidcr.nih.gov/oralhealth/Topics/TMJ/TMJDisorders.htm

Stressed Out? Your Teeth are Probably Feeling the Pressure

"I sheared off my front tooth," actor Demi Moore explained to *Tonight Show* host Jimmy Fallon during a show back in June 2017.

"I'd love to say it was skateboarding or something really kind of cool, but I think it's something that's important to share because I think it's literally, probably after heart disease, one of the biggest killers in America, which is stress."[31]

While stress doesn't immediately cause your teeth to fracture, loosen, or fall out, it can cause this kind of damage over time, with stress increasingly becoming more prevalent in younger generations.[32] Under high stress, people may forget to brush or floss, and may not have the time or even think to visit the dentist. The same conditions can also lead to increased cortisol levels in the body, and while cortisol in the short term has an anti-inflammatory effect, extended or exaggerated stress response can lead to cortisol dysfunction, which can result in widespread inflammation and pain.

Stress in America—Harder on Young Adults

According to the American Psychological Association (APA), stress is becoming more of an issue for younger generations (Millennials born between 1984 and 2004, and Gen-Xers born between 1964 and 1984), who report feeling the most stress and the least relief compared to older generations. As of the APA's 2015 stress survey, adults in America:

- Report stress levels higher than what they believe is healthy (3.8 on a 10 point scale)

---

31 Bruce Lee, "Demi Moore Lost Two Teeth To Stress, Here's How It Can Happen," Forbes, last modified June 15, 2017, https://www.forbes.com/sites/brucelee/2017/06/15/demi-moore-lost-two-teeth-to-stress-heres-how-it-can-happen/

32 "2015 Stress in America," American Psychological Association, http://www.apa.org/news/press/releases/stress/2015/snapshot.aspx

- Rate their average stress level as 5.1 on a 10 point scale (up from 4.9 in 2014)
- Were more likely to report experiencing at least one symptom of stress (78 percent vs. 74 percent in 2014)
- Were more likely to report experiencing extreme stress (24 percent vs. 18 percent in 2014)
- Reported higher incidences of illness, with:
  - 67 percent receiving a diagnosis of at least one chronic illness
  - 16 percent diagnosed with depression (up from 12 percent)
  - 13 percent with anxiety disorder (up from 9 percent) 32 percent with high blood pressure (up from 24 percent)
  - 58 percent with obesity
- Millennials and Gen-Xers were more likely to rate money as a stress source
- 45 percent of Millennials say their stress levels have increased in the past year
- 39 percent of Gen-Xers say their stress levels have increased in the past year
- Young adults are more likely than other generations to engage in stress coping/management activities, yet one in four young adults say they don't feel they're doing enough to manage their stress.

Stress can also lead to bruxism, which is the medical term for teeth grinding. If you apply enough force to your teeth, over a long enough period of time, you can do significant damage. On average, a human can bite down with two hundred pounds of force per square inch, which is actually pretty powerful, and when you apply that kind force regularly on just about anything, it's going to cause some damage.

To understand how that kind of pressure affects the mouth, consider how this part of the body is composed. The tissues surrounding the teeth, for instance, are basically tight strands similar to guitar strings, holding everything together. But when you put excessive pressure on guitar strings, what happens? They pop, which is basically what is happening to the tissues around your teeth when you clench and grind. This is why the gums start to recede around teeth affected by bruxism, as the forces cause those tissues to break. If those forces continue, they go on to wear away the enamel, exposing the dentin and creating access points for bacteria to get directly into the blood stream.

Bruxism can occur consciously or subconsciously, while you're awake or asleep, and may not seem to be a concern for months or even years after it first starts to occur.

Signs of bruxism include:

- Dull headaches (especially in the morning)

- Sore jaw muscles

- Pain radiating from the ear

- Teeth sensitivity

- Chipped, cracked teeth

- Loose teeth

- Damage on the inside of the cheek from chewing or biting

- Indentations in the tongue

While bruxism is common in younger children, the condition is usually temporary and more likely due to allergies, teething, or misaligned baby teeth as opposed to stress. Most children outgrow teeth grinding by their teens.

If bruxism continues, or if you suffer from it as an adult, then the long-term pressure and grinding of the teeth can lead to chipping, cracks, and loose teeth that may eventually fall out, as well as the wearing down of the enamel. In severe cases, the enamel can become so worn that the underlying layer of dentin is exposed. This not only causes sensitivity, but the dentin, which is nine times softer than enamel, is much more susceptible to decay.

In rare cases, long-term bruxing can lead to the enlargement of facial muscles, which can block the salivary glands, leading to swelling, pain, inflammation, and dry mouth. And dry mouth alone is a major trigger for cavity formation as the lack of saliva means that the mouth doesn't have its natural means of regular cleansing available to it.

While stress can certainly result in bruxism, teeth grinding can also be related to sleep issues or any of those childhood conditions listed earlier, such as a misaligned bite or allergies. In milder cases, bruxism may not necessarily need treatment. But if the problem persists to the point of discomfort, jaw pain, and damage to the teeth, then one or multiple forms of treatment may be recommended.

Treating Teeth Grinding (Bruxism)

Dental treatment

Although dental treatment may help to relieve the effect of bruxism, it won't necessarily treat the cause. Some options include:

- **Mouth guards and occlusal splints**: mouth guards can protect your teeth from grinding directly against each other while you sleep, and occlusal splints can be custom built to keep your teeth in an ideal bite position, as well as prevent direct contact of teeth during sleep.

- **Dental correction**: if the degree of bruxism has lead to teeth becoming so sensitive that you can no longer drink hot or cold liquids or chew properly, then the teeth may need to be reshaped and restored in order to repair the damage.

Behavior modification

If stress is a likely cause of bruxism, behavioral medication and management may help:

- **Stress management**: learning strategies that promote relaxation such as meditation, may help to reduce anxiety, which may have a positive impact on bruxism.

- **Behavior modification**: if you're aware of bruxism and how it's manifesting in your jaw habits, then you may be able to change that behavior by practicing proper jaw positioning, as demonstrated by your dentist.

- **Biofeedback**: through the use of electrical sensors, you can view information on how your body is reacting to subtle changes, which may help in reducing those actions that result in bruxing. For instance, learning how to consciously control your breathing and heart rate can be a helpful calming technique, and learning how to effectively relax the mouth and jaw muscles may reduce the effects of bruxism, or help to eliminate it altogether if it's main source is stress and muscle tension.

- **Lifestyle modifications**: some at-home methods for reducing the factors that contribute to bruxism can include:

  □ Taking relaxing baths, listening to soothing music or exercising

  □ Avoiding stimulating substances such as alcohol or coffee in the evening

  □ Getting a good nights sleep

  □ Asking your sleep partner to let you know if they hear you making any grinding noises, or if your jaw is clicking at night, so you can inform your dentist or doctor

  □ Schedule regular dental exams to spot signs of bruxism early

By addressing teeth grinding earlier in life, you're more likely to avoid its longer-term impacts, and more likely to make it into your later years with most, if not all, of your natural teeth.

Retaining that Smile

While this book isn't meant to focus on only orthodontics, a lot of what happens as part of your orthodontist visits directly affect your dentist visits, and vice versa.

For instance, if you had braces as a teenager, it's likely that your dentist played an important part in keeping your teeth clean between orthodontist visits, and reporting any concerns, breaks or other conditions to your orthodontist.

After the braces come off, that relationship between orthodontist, dentist and patient continues as the patient is monitored to ensure that the braces did what they were intended to do—and a big part of that has to do with whether or not the patient is good about wearing a retainer.

It's a tough ask for a teenager who just got out of braces to continue wearing another appliance, but the first year after braces is vital for ensuring that the teeth are secure in their new locations. This is why we likely recommend that you wear your retainer up to twenty-two hours every day for the first year, then every night for the following two years. Most kids are pretty good about that extra year—its the time afterward that presents the most challenge.

If you wore braces as a kid, you should still be wearing your retainer at least three nights a week and ideally every night for the rest of your life.

This is because, even with all of that time in braces, your teeth are going to shift. It may take a couple decades, but your teeth will gradually shift forward and inward with age—unless you have gingivitis or periodontal disease, in which case your teeth will shift much sooner than that.

If, by chance, you have been wearing your retainer regularly since your teenage years, then the other caveat of maintaining that healthy straight smile is getting your retainer replaced as needed; every two to ten years, depending on how rough you are on them. This isn't just because the retainer can wear out, however—it's also because of the inevitable tooth drift that occurs as you get older. Even with retention, teeth are going to shift slightly and the retainer will need to be adjusted in order to keep those teeth in proper alignment. And if you need a new set and you no longer live near your old orthodontist, don't worry— any orthodontist can have a new one made for you.

Over the course of a lifetime, you may go through several retainers, but wearing a retainer at night a few nights out of the week is a small price to pay for the long-term benefit of keeping your teeth straight and healthy.

Chapter Eleven

AGES 40–59

For most of us, that feeling of invincibility that we've had our whole lives is likely starting to wear off in this stage—and our systems are starting to wind down a little along with it.

On the brighter side, this is the stage of life where a lot of us start taking better care of our bodies. Before this age, parents in particular were putting their children's health ahead of their own, making sure the kids went to the doctor and dentist regularly while neglecting their own health. Once the kids start to grow up, however—and in some cases move out of the house—moms and dads start to reinvest in making themselves look and feel better, working on getting their looks as close to—or better than—they were in their pre-kid days. This likely means more working out and more time at the dentist, looking into what can not only be done health-wise but also cosmetically.

Unfortunately, this is also the age when people who were neglecting the signs and symptoms of gingivitis are now likely suffering from full-on periodontal disease.

What is Periodontal Disease (Periodontitis)?

Periodontal disease occurs when gingivitis isn't treated, and the gums pull away from the teeth, forming spaces that then become infected. In fact, the word "periodontitis" means "inflammation around the tooth." As the infection grows, the toxins and the immune system begin to break down the bone and tissues holding the infected teeth in place, eventually leading to tooth loss.

The signs and symptoms of periodontal disease are the same as gingivitis—as are the risk factors. Treatment, too, follows the same path, beginning with a complete deep cleaning that involves scraping the tartar from above and below the gum line, and removing rough spots on the tooth root where germs gather. In some cases, a laser may be used to remove all of the offending buildup.

Antibiotic and antimicrobial medications may also be recommended after a deep cleaning, but if the damage is too extensive, surgery is most likely the next step.

Surgical Treatments for Periodontal Disease

There are two main types of surgical procedures for periodontal disease. Depending on the extent of the damage, your dentist may recommend:

Flap Surgery

This procedure involves lifting back the gums to remove extensive tartar deposits, followed by suturing the gums back into place so that everything fits tightly. Once healed, the gums should fit snug around the tooth and the teeth may appear longer as a result.

Bone & Tissue Grafts

Sometimes flap surgery isn't enough, however, particularly when the disease has eaten away at the gum tissue and even the bone underneath. Bone grafting involves placing a piece of natural or synthetic bone in the area of bone loss in order to stimulate growth. In some cases, guided tissue regeneration may also be used, which involves placing a piece of mesh between the gum and bone that blocks the gum tissue from growing where the bone should be, giving the bone and connective tissue time to grow. A graft of soft tissue may also be used for gum loss, with synthetic material or tissue from another part of the mouth being used to cover exposed tooth roots.

The success of either procedure is entirely dependent on the patient, his or her risk factors and how well mouth health is maintained at home going forward.[33]

Believe it or not, one out of every two Americans over the age of thirty have some stage of periodontitis. And in adults over the age of sixty-five, the prevalence is a little over 70 percent of all Americans.[34]

---

33 "Periodontal (Gum) Disease: Causes, Symptoms, and Treatments," National Institute of Dental and Craniofacial Research, last modified September 2013, https://www.nidcr.nih.gov/OralHealth/Topics/GumDiseases/PeriodontalGumDisease.htm

34 "CDC: Half of American Adults Have Periodontal Disease," American Academy of Periodontology, https://www.perio.org/consumer/cdc-study.htm

Half of American Adults have Periodontal Disease

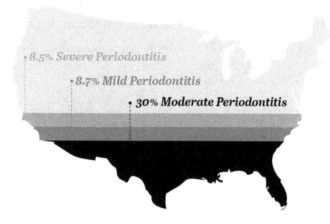

- 8.5% *Severe Periodontitis*
- 8.7% *Mild Periodontitis*
- 30% *Moderate Periodontitis*

47.2% of American Adults have Periodontitis,

that's **64.7 Million** Adults 30 years and older

Source: American Academy of Periodontology/Centers for Disease Control

Interestingly enough, according to a study conducted in part by the Centers for Disease Control (CDC), men are more likely than women to have periodontal disease (56.4 percent vs. 38.4 percent in women), and those at the highest risk include current smokers (64.2 percent), those with less than a high school education (66.9 percent) and those living below the federal poverty level (65.4 percent).

"Periodontal disease is associated with age," stated Paul Eke, MPH, PhD, lead author of the study and CDC epidemiologist, "and as Americans live longer and retain more of their natural teeth, periodontal disease may take on more prominence in the oral health of the U.S. Adult population. Maintaining good periodontal health is important to the overall health and well-being of our aging population."

With these findings, co-author Robert Genco, DDS, PhD, believes that periodontal disease should be elevated to the level of Public Health Concern. "We now know that periodontal disease is one of the most prevalent, non-communicable chronic diseases in our population, similar to cardiovascular disease and diabetes," Genco stated.[35]

Have You Had Your Annual Comprehensive Periodontal Evaluation?

According to the American Academy of Periodontology, every dental patient should have a comprehensive periodontal evaluation conducted on annual basis to gauge periodontal health, diagnose existing disease, assess risk for disease, and determine any needed treatment. This service can be conducted during a regular dental visit by the general dentist, or by a dental hygienist or periodontist.

Crowning Moment

If you've had cavities since you were a kid, then crowns are very likely in your near future. Between the ages of forty and sixty is when most fillings have run their effective course. If you've been keeping up with your dental visits, then a cavity that you had filled in your pre-teens or teens was likely redone in your twenties or early thirties. Depending on the original size of the cavity, the redo of that filling will likely take away sig-nificantly more of the surrounding structure. Then,

---

35   P.I. Eke et al., "Prevalence of Periodontitis in Adults in the United States: 2009 and 2010," *Journal of Dental Research* 91, no. 10 (August 2012), https://doi.org/10.1177/0022034512457373

when the cavity needs to be replaced again in, say, ten to fifteen years, then there's a good chance that there won't be enough tooth structure left for a filling, and a crown will need to be placed instead.

The fact of the matter is that if you have a cavity, you're going to end up with a crown. It might be sooner, if the cavity is bigger or if you are particularly rough on your teeth, or it might be later—but it's almost always necessary.

Snoring Problem or Obstructive Sleep Apnea?

While obstructive sleep apnea can occur at any age, the risk factor increases with age and the condition is more prevalent in men over the age of forty. While this may not seem like a condition that you would immediately think to bring up with your dentist, we're actually in one of the best positions to help with this disorder as treatment often involves adjusting the jaw in order to open up the airway and increase airflow.

Obstructive sleep apnea, or OSA, is a medical condition in which the sufferer stops breathing for seconds up to minutes at a time while sleeping. These pauses in breathing, called "apneas," can occur thirty or more times in an hour, and breathing often starts again with a loud choking sound or snort. This disruption may not entirely wake the person up, but it will move them from a deep sleep to a light slight sleep, which greatly reduces the overall quality of their sleep and leads to excessive daytime sleepiness.

Even though OSA is a common condition, it often goes undiagnosed as those who suffer from it don't realize it's occurring unless someone tells them. And if a sleep partner does notice, they often write it off as loud snoring instead of something more. If you're concerned that someone is suffering from OSA, the best way to tell is by listening for that pause in breathing between snores. Snoring is usually only a split-second closure of the upper airway that doesn't interrupt the sleeper, while OSA sufferers will noticeably stop breathing before starting again.

Along with that audible pause, other signs and symptoms of the condition include:

- excessive sleepiness

- fatigue

- memory impairment

- mood disturbance

- decreased libido

- social withdrawal

- cardiovascular disease

- lower jaw is too small or is set too far back

- presence of hypertension

- BMI of 30 or higher

- neck circumference of 17 inches or larger

- observed choking or gasping during sleep

- inattention and changes in energy levels during the day

- enlarged tonsils and/or adenoids

There is also evidence that people who suffer from bruxism— teeth grinding—may also have some degree of OSA as that jaw movement may be related to the subconscious effort to keep the airway open during sleep, moving the jaw around or clenching it in order to activate the throat and neck muscles and keep the airway open.

Diagnosing Obstructive Sleep Apnea

The method for determining if someone is suffering from sleep apnea is typically two parts: a basic sleep screening followed by a sleep study conducted with a polysomnograph, or PSG.

The sleep screening can be conducted at the dentist office and usually involves a series of questions or situations to determine someone's daytime sleepiness scale. Two of the more well known surveys are the Epworth Sleepiness Questionnaire and the Berlin Questionnaire.

Questions on these tests might include gauging the chances that you'll doze off (not feel tired) in situations such as:

- Watching television

- Sitting and reading

- Sitting inactive in a public place such as a meeting

- As a passenger in a car for longer than one continuous hour

- Sitting and talking to someone

- Sitting quietly after a lunch without alcohol

- In a car while stopped for traffic

Other evaluative methods include assessing sleep habits as well as taking physical factors into account, as is the case with the STOP-BANG Questionnaire, with the name of the test standing for "snoring, tired, observed pressure, body mass index, age, neck circumference, and gender."

Additional evaluation methods could include a cephalometric analysis, to identify any growth abnormalities that may be affecting breathing, a Cone Beam CT Analysis to measure minimum airway volume, an intraoral evaluation to check for any potential visible obstructions, or a take home sleep monitor to measure key parameters like blood oxygen saturation, apnea and hypopnea episodes, and disturbed breathing patterns.

If one or more of these screenings do confirm the risk of OSA, the next step is a supervised sleep study monitored by a polysomnograph (PSG).

While a PSG will measure dozens of factors while the patient is sleeping, one of the most important factors it will be measuring is the person's apnea-hypopnea index, or AHI. This measurement determines exactly how many apneas, or pauses in breathing, the patient experiences in an hour, as well as moments of shallow breathing called "hypopneas". Additionally, the study will count the number of respiratory effort-related arousals the patient experiences within an hour's time.

These measurements, along with accounts of the patient's heart rate, airflow, air pressure in the esophagus, oxygen saturation, snoring, eye movement, and even carbon dioxide levels of the skin, are taken into account before presenting the patient with a diagnosis.

Treating Obstructive Sleep Apnea

This is where dentists can play a significant role in treating or even curing OSA. If the condition is caused by a restricted airway, then the patient may benefit from oral appliance therapy.

There are several options for oral appliances that help with sleep apnea, and all of them are designed to hold the lower jaw forward, which creates a larger space between the base of the tongue and the back of the throat. If a patient is experiencing constriction at night, this adjustment should help keep that area more clear.

However, since oral appliances generally rely on the teeth to do their job, they're not recommended for people with periodontal disease or TMJ issues, as the appliance may exacerbate the condition. There are also potential side effects of long term usage, including:

- dry mouth

- excessive salivation

- tooth discomfort

- gingival irritation

- jaw muscle tenderness

- TMJ discomfort

- changes in bite due to teeth shifting from the pressure placed on them by the appliance. *

*This last side effect can often be managed by wearing a tooth positioner—a device that resembles a large sports mouth guard—for twenty to thirty minutes per day to keep the patients' teeth in their original position.

If oral appliances aren't an option, then the most common treatment for the condition is a continuous positive airway pressure device, or CPAP, which blows compressed air into the patient's nose and/or mouth while sleeping. While the CPAP is considered the "gold standard" for OSA treatment, it's also the least tolerated, as the mask can be uncomfortable to wear, and the pressure on the airway can irritate the nasal and upper airway tissues. Other options for treating sleep apnea, apart from lifestyle and behavior modification (losing weight, avoiding sleeping on the back, avoiding alcohol and/ or sedatives before bed, etc), may include:

- **Upper airway electrical stimulation**: a device that can be implanted in the chest to deliver mild electrical impulses to the nerve that controls the tongue, stimulating it to move when the patient stops breathing.

- **Maxillomandibular (double-jaw) advancement surgery**: for patients with significantly narrow airways, surgically moving the upper and lower jaws forward can help to open up the airway and tighten the muscles and tendons in those airways, reducing the risk of airway collapse.

- **Tonsillectomy and Adenoidectomy**: patients presenting with sleep apnea during childhood are more likely to benefit from these procedures, and have been shown to be highly effective in treating pediatric OSA.

- **Tracheostomy**: this procedure creates a small opening in the trachea below an obstruction in the airway. This procedure is usually only done in extreme cases of OSA, when no other options are available.

- **Nasal procedures**: if sleep apnea is mainly due to restrictions in the nasal area, surgeries can be conducted to address the blockage.

- **Uvulopalatopharyngoplasty**: This is a big word for an interesting procedure, which involves removing a portion of the soft palate around the uvula (that fleshy tissue hanging down in the back of the mouth) in order to open up the airway. While this can help with snoring, however, it's typically not as effective as other surgeries and therapies for treating OSA.

Now is the best time for preventative dental care

It never hurts to remind yourself that your dental health down the road depends on how healthy you keep your teeth today. As you age, any problems you have today are going to get worse unless they're treated, and neglect today can result in new issues and problems tomorrow. Overall health can go downhill fast, and keeping your mouth young in old age requires diligence; brushing and flossing twice a day are more important than ever, and keeping regular dental appointments will ultimately cost you much less in the long run, as failing to see the dentist could mean bigger—and costlier—dental conditions down the road.

In addition, remember those conditions that have been linked in one way or another to overall mouth health—diabetes, heart disease, stroke and respiratory problems have all been tied to the risk of bacteria from gum infections slipping directly into the bloodstream and triggering inflammation in organs and tissues.

Want to make it into your golden years with as many of your own, real teeth as possible? Then today is the best day to start a proper dental care routine that will last you the rest of your life.

Chapter Twelve

AGES 60+

Cavities and lost teeth are a serious issue at this age, in part due to the long-term wear and tear on gums and teeth that has already taken place.

With an average bite of two hundred pounds of pressure per square inch, the human mouth is pretty powerful, but that power also has the ability to wear down on the outer layer of tooth enamel over time. And when you combine a lifetime of chewing and grinding along with exposure to damaging acidic foods and drinks, you run the risk of more cracks, breaks, cavities and overall damage due to that weakened enamel.[36]

---

36 "The aging mouth – and how to keep it younger," Harvard Health Publishing, Harvard Medical School, last modified January 2010, https://www.health.harvard.edu/diseases-and-conditions/the-aging-mouth-and-how-to-keep-it-younger

Gum recession, too, is more common in older adults, with a little more than 70 percent of people over the age of fifty showing some degree of recession, and 90 percent with signs of recession over the age of eighty.[37] When this condition is left untreated, the exposed root is more susceptible to gum disease, which could eventually lead to the destruction of the gum tissue and even the bone around the teeth.

Although there's not much you can do to stop the natural wearing down of tooth enamel, keeping up with daily dental health habits such as brushing, flossing, and regular dental visits are as important as ever at this age.

Toothbrushing a Challenge? Go Electric!

Daily habits that we used to do without a thought can become more burdensome in our later years. Just brushing teeth, for instance, can be difficult if arthritis or other disabilities affecting motor skills are beginning to manifest. For those with limited dexterity, switching from a manual toothbrush to an electric one can make a big difference. Additionally, switching to fluoride toothpastes that aid in the remineralization of the teeth can help strengthen tooth enamel and fill in the weak areas that plaque tends to cling to.

Dry Mouth (xerostomia)

Because of the prevalence of medications being taken in this age range, for conditions ranging from diabetes to blood pressure to cancer treatment, dry mouth is a common occurrence. Not only does this usually result in bad breath, but the lack of the mouth's natural cleanser—saliva—means that cavities are starting to come back into

---

37 Claudia Hammond, "Is age the cause of receding gums?" BBC Future, last modified August 7, 2013, http://www.bbc.com/future/story/20130807-does-age-damage-your-gums

play, and habits to combat the condition, such as sucking on sugary cough drops or hard candies, aren't helping the situation.

Dry mouth can also be a problem for denture wearers, as the lack of saliva can make the dentures feel loose in the mouth, leading to discomfort. In these cases, a denture fixative and/or artificial saliva can help, as can drinking sips of water frequently throughout the day. Other options for combating dry mouth include:

- Chewing sugarless gum

- Sucking on sugarless candies

- Avoiding alcohol or caffeinated beverages

- Avoiding tobacco

Varnish for a Healthier Smile

Even though cavities may seem like something only kids have to worry about, the fact is that the rate of tooth decay for people ages sixty-five-plus is now exceeding the rate of cavities in schoolchildren.[38] Part of this is due to those two age-related conditions mentioned earlier: dry mouth and gum recession. As the lack of self-cleaning saliva becomes more prevalent and more of that soft root tissue becomes exposed, the risk of developing cavities increases, particularly along the gum line.

To get ahead of that risk, more dentists are beginning to recommend a fluoride varnish around the base, or neck, of the teeth. The varnish, which usually consists of anywhere between .1 percent and 5 percent sodium fluoride and a resin or synthetic base that helps it stick to the teeth, sets rapidly and can be applied quickly, reducing

---

38 "The aging mouth – and how to keep it younger," Harvard Health Publishing, Harvard Medical School, last modified January 2010, https://www.health.harvard. edu/diseases-and-conditions/the-aging-mouth-and-how-to-keep-it-younger

the time that the hygienist spends in the mouth and minimizing the risk of gagging or accidental swallowing of the product.

While the majority of studies into the effectiveness of fluoride varnishes in preventing cavities have been conducted on children, more researchers are beginning to look into its impact on older adults. For children, systematic reviews have proven how effective topical fluoride can be in preventing or slowing the progress of cavities. With older adults, recent reviews have also shown a reduction in root cavities, with fluoride varnish controlling root cavities better than brushing with a high fluoride toothpaste alone. The study concluded that fluoride varnishes on older adults, particularly those who have difficulty brushing, would benefit from varnish being applied to the base of the teeth three to four times a year.[39]

Dental Implants and Dentures

More and more, implants are becoming the norm over dentures when it comes to replacing missing teeth. There are multiple reasons why— the main one being that implants look and act like real teeth. This doesn't just mean being able to tear into a corn-on-the-cob anytime you want—it also applies to how the implant acts in the mouth.

With dentures, the offending teeth are removed from the mouth and nothing replaces them. Over time, the body reabsorbs the bone that the teeth were removed from since it's no longer supporting teeth, leading to the degradation and thinning of the jaw. Implants, however, are made with a material that bonds with the bone, acting like real teeth so that the body isn't stimulated to begin reabsorption.

---

39   Nicola Innes and Dafydd Evans, "Caries prevention for older people in residential care homes," *Evidence-Based Dentistry* 10, no. 3 (2009): 83–87, https://doi.org/10.1038/sj.ebd.6400672

Other benefits include comfort—implants act like real teeth instead of shifting in the mouth or requiring fixatives, as dentures do—and longevity. The typical implant has a failure rate of less than 5 percent and lasts an average of twenty-five years, with some said to last a lifetime. Meanwhile, the lifecycle of dentures is usually anywhere from seven to fifteen years.[40]

Implants are also a healthier option for the surrounding teeth, as well. When a bridge is placed, for instance, the two teeth adjacent to the area need to be ground down so they can hold the bridge structure. Consequently, these newly worn teeth are more vulnerable to decay and damage.

How are Implants Implanted?

The implant procedure typically involves placing a titanium screw in just the right place in the jawbone, followed by the attachment of the prosthetic tooth. In some cases, patients may opt for a combination of implant and denture, in which a series of titanium screws are implanted in the jaw, with the external end shaped so that a partial or full denture can be snapped onto it.

Implants don't work for all patients, however. If you smoke, have diabetes, or have substantial bone loss already, implants may not be the best option.

What to Know Before Whitening Older Teeth

As the outer layer of enamel thins, the dentin underneath becomes more visible, making teeth appear less white. Coffee, red wine, tea,

---

40   Lesley Alderman, "For Most, Implants Beat Dentures, but at a Price," Health, The New York Times, last modified July 30, 2010, http://www.nytimes.com/2010/07/31/health/31patient.html

and tobacco can also stain teeth, leading them to potentially look older than they are.

While over-the-counter whitening products and whitening toothpastes can help lighten teeth by a few shades, the effects are often much less dramatic in older teeth. However, before going through with a full-on dental whitening, keep in mind that professional whitening procedures may leave teeth feeling more sensitive and some stains may be more challenging to remove than others, requiring several rounds of bleaching before they can be removed.

Are Teeth Affected by Osteoporosis?

Osteoporosis, a medical condition that decreases the density of bones and makes them more likely to fracture, can also affect the bone density in the mouth. According to a study by the National Institute of Health, women with osteoporosis were three times more likely to have a loose tooth than women without the condition.[41]

Watching Out for Signs of Oral Cancer

As is the case with most cancers, the risk of oral cancer increases with age and the use of tobacco products. With each year that someone smokes or chews tobacco, the risk of developing oral cancer increases.

When oral cancer does develop, it's most likely to develop on the lower lip first, followed by the upper lip and then the tongue. Initial signs and symptoms of the disease are easy to miss, but if you notice a white or red patch on your lip, tongue, or bottom of your mouth that lasts longer than two weeks, let your dentist know about it. While it may be the early signs of oral cancer, there's also the chance that

---

41   "Oral Health and Bone Disease," NIH Osteoporosis and Related Bone Diseases National Resource Center, https://www.bones.nih.gov/health-info/bone/bone-health/oral-health/oral-health-and-bone-disease

it could be a sore caused by herpes or yeast infection, which, while painful, can also be treated.

Dental Care and Dementia

Older adults suffering from forms of dementia such as Alzheimer's disease should be allowed to conduct their own dental care for as long as they can, with reminders from family and caregivers, and supervision if needed. Establishing a daily care routine in the early stages of dementia is particularly important as assistance in brushing teeth may be needed later on.

Since it can often be challenging to communicate with someone who has dementia, it may be hard to tell if that person is suffering from mouth pain or discomfort. If you're a caregiver or family member of someone with dementia, it can help to keep an eye out for the following signs of potential dental problems:

- Refusing to eat hot or cold foods, or any food

- Frequent pulling at the face and mouth

- Increased moaning, shouting, or restlessness

- Refusal to take part in daily activities

- Aggressive behavior

- Disturbed sleep

- Not wearing dentures[42]

---

42 "Dental Care," Alzheimer's Society, https://www.alzheimers.org.uk/info/20029/daily_living/9/dental_care/3

Dental Treatment for those Suffering from Dementia

According to the Alzheimer's Society, dental treatment for those suffering from dementia should be considered with all of the stages of dementia in mind. During the early stages, for instance, dentists should recommend and conduct treatment with the understanding that the patient will not be able to care for his or her own teeth at some point. Therefore, preventative treatments for conditions such as gum disease are very important. As the disease progresses, patients may need sedation or general anesthesia for dental visits, and their ability to co-operate during these visits should be assessed beforehand. In the late stages of dementia, the challenges of thinking clearly along with physical frailty and often additional complex medical conditions can make dental visits challenging, and care should mainly focus on maintaining the patient's comfort, preventing dental disease, and providing emergency treatment.[43]

When considering dental treatment for dementia patients, the following factors should be kept in mind:

- What dental problems are being experienced

- Whether the patient is able to give informed consent

- The patient's level of independence, thinking abilities, physical impairments, co-operation and mental state.

Once these conditions are assessed, the dentist can provide input on the best treatment options for the patient, and how regularly he or she should see the dentist.

As with every stage of life, keeping teeth in their best condition requires regular maintenance and common sense practices. With this

---

43   Ibid.

in mind, a little effort now can make a big difference in the teeth you get to keep—and their overall health—down the road.

For more information, or if you would like to schedule an appointment for a complimentary examination, please call us at (833)-OCCSmiles, contact us by email at info@OCCSmiles.com, or visit our website at www.OCCSmiles.com.

Printed in the USA
CPSIA information can be obtained
at www.ICGtesting.com
JSHW012039140824
68134JS00033B/3145